D1549511

615. 321

The Healing art

615 . 321

HEALING ART OF HERBS

Books should be returned or renewed by the last
date stamped above.

NP56

THE HEALING ART OF
HERBS

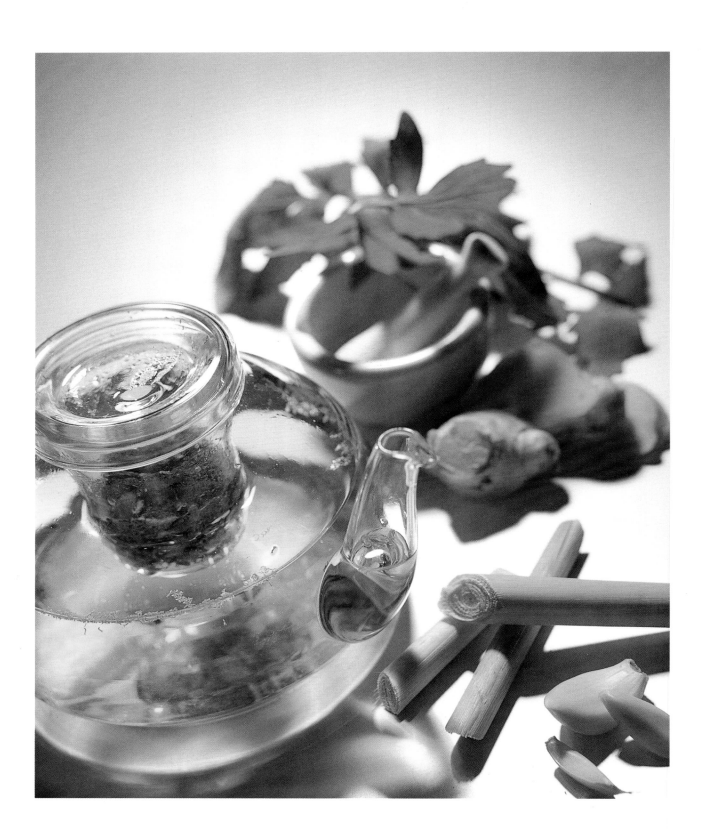

THE HEALING ART OF
HERBS

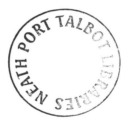

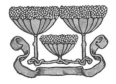

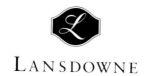

LANSDOWNE

Contents

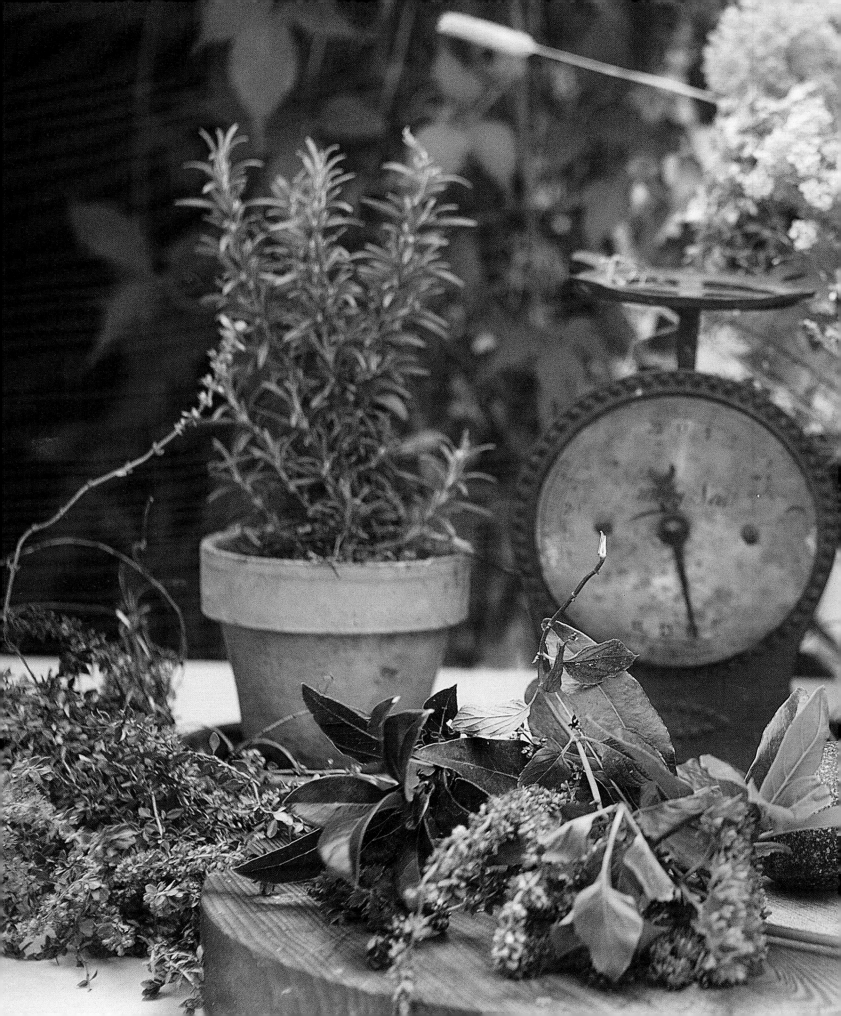

Introduction to Herbs

You can learn how to use herbs and herbal treatments to enliven your diet, beautify and purify your body, and calm your mind.

Knowledge of herbs was acquired in ancient times through sometimes dangerous trial and error. In recent decades, sophisticated investigation of the chemical and biological properties of herbs has extended that knowledge. Still, our ignorance on the subject of herbs exceeds our knowledge. Scientists estimate that 90 per cent of the organic constituents of the half million species of plants growing throughout the world are yet to be identified.

We do have at our disposal a valuable store of herbal information, however, in the extraordinary library of herbals which documents the use of plants in everyday life throughout the world and over thousands of years.

The simplicity and gentle action of herbal treatments and remedies appeal to people in this century of high-tech conventional medicine, expensively packaged cosmetics, and food adulterated with artificial additives.

Often the same herbs our ancestors used can be found today growing vigorously by the roadside, on vacant building sites, as well as in rural or wilderness areas. But for convenience sake, many people prefer to cultivate their own herbs.

Most herbs are simple to grow, harvest, store, and use. Many herbs encourage the micro-organisms which keep fruit, vegetable, and flower gardens free from plant pests and diseases; and indoors, herbs will discourage many common household pests. Herbs used medicinally produce an effective result in a healthy way, without the unpleasant and harmful side effects which sometimes accompany modern pharmaceuticals. We can also use herbs to safely and economically enhance the food we eat or beautify our bodies.

It is simple and inexpensive to enjoy different herbs: mint plucked from the kitchen garden will make a tea to calm an upset stomach; nurture marigolds and enjoy the sight of their bright gold faces as they follow the sun's daily transit. And when you brush past basil, thyme, or chamomile their distinctive scents are released into the atmosphere creating moments of particular pleasure.

But you don't have to be a gardener to enjoy the benefits of herbs in modern life. A great variety of fresh and dried herbs are now readily available on the shelves of supermarkets, health food stores, and other specialty outlets. Several companies produce high quality herbal treatments, medicinal or cosmetic, at competitive prices, and there are numerous well-qualified herbalists to guide you in their use.

And if, as the old adage has it, prevention is better than cure, consider the sense of wellbeing, in itself conducive to good health, which is experienced by the many people who bring herbs into their lives. It is surely a reminder to us of the fundamentally beneficial value of plants.

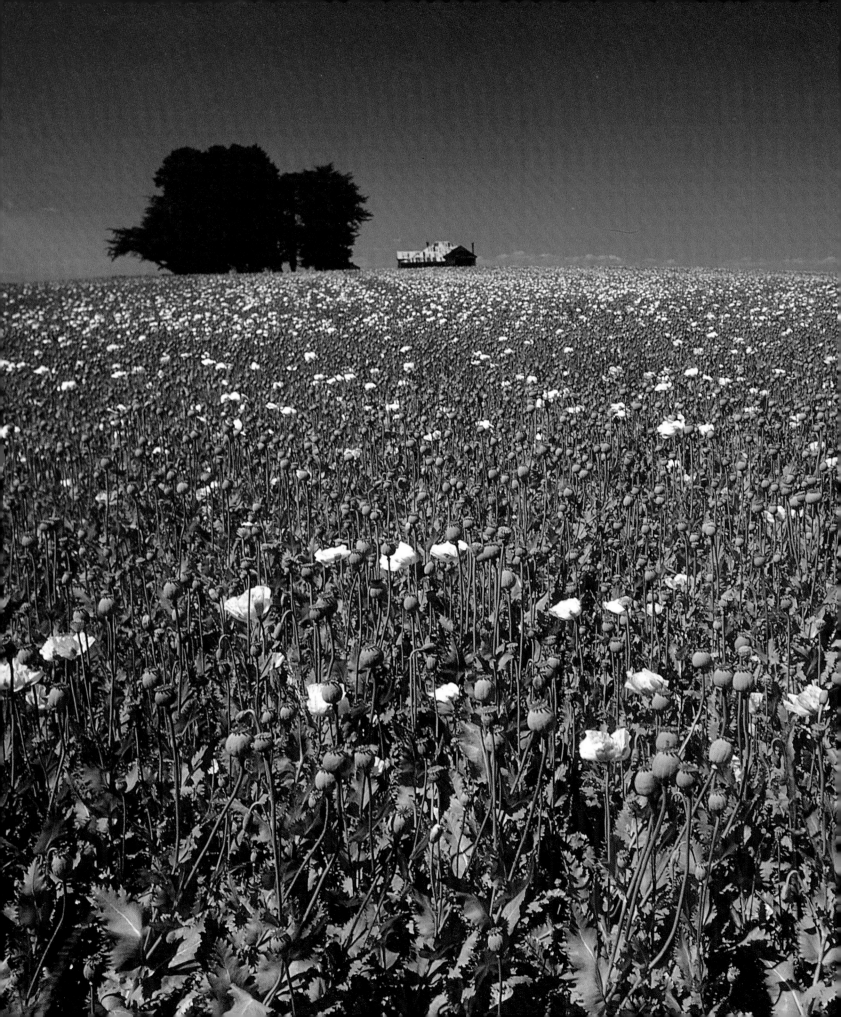

Herbalism in History

The history of herbalism is a fascinating and dramatic one, interwoven with the social, political, and economic structures of communities throughout the world.

The original practitioners of herbal medicine were usually women, the predominant gatherers of food in early tribal groups. Herbs were among the plants they harvested as food, or as building or clothing materials.

Tribal women herbalists experimented with plant life native to their territory, exploring the mysteries of herbs in relation to health and ill-health. Generations of trial and error taught them which plants were good for treating illness, which were good to eat, and which would cause poisoning and death. In their caves and rough shelters, they administered the first herbal treatments: crushed leaves, seeds or berries, saps, oils, and juices to comfort and heal the stricken. The women handed their knowledge down to their daughters and on to subsequent generations of female custodians to further benefit their societies.

Because tribes thrived or perished according to the seasons and the occurrence of natural phenomena, these early societies believed the world was controlled by supernatural forces. Men with their greater physical power assumed the roles of chiefs and shamans (priests who interceded between gods and humans), while women continued their experiments with the healing art of herbs. Disease of body or mind was attributed to the power of malevolent spirits; but with the gain of herbal knowledge came a keen observation of the natural world, and a belief developed that herbs had effects not only on the physical, but on the invisible aspects of human beings. While women administered their herbal remedies to the sick, the shaman smoked or ingested hallucinogens inducing a trancelike state. From here, he would seek out the spirit of the ailing individual which he would cure on the spirit plane.

Written records of herbal study date back over 5,000 years to the Sumerians. A herbal from China, dating around 2700 BC lists 365 medicinal plants. The earliest Ayurvedic texts from India date from around 2500 BC. This medicine, like that of the ancient Greeks, sees illness in terms of an imbalance of the humors and seeks to rectify this using herbs and dietary control. Additional herbal traditions came with the Persian invasions of 500 BC and in the fourteenth century, the Moguls brought Galenic medicine to India.

Herbal knowledge has largely survived into the present day, despite the indiscriminate destruction of books and the halt to learning that characterized the Dark Ages, and the periodic persecutions and purges of those village wise women who tended gardens and used herbal skills to heal and strengthen their communities.

Among the earliest successes of herbal medicine are those recorded in the history of Ancient Egypt. The great healer, Imhotep, physician to King Djoser of the Third Dynasty (3000 BC), was so revered that he came to be regarded as a god. The ingredients of medical prescriptions used by doctors in ancient Egypt came from the medical papyri compiled during the period 1500-1000 BC. The ingredients came mainly from plants and trees and their fruits. Many of these have medicinal properties recognized in modern herbal medicine. Like our medicines, when a remedy was prescribed by a doctor, it came in a labelled bottle. This papyri was for the use of the medical profession; the housewife had to rely on experience and approximate measurements.

Myths throughout the world record both mystical and physical properties of herbs. An Egyptian myth tells of the goddess Isis concocting a poultice of coriander, juniper berries, wormwood, and honey to cure a headache for the god Ea. Isis was the Egyptian goddess of the earth and its fruits, the Nile, the sea, the underworld, love, healing, and magic. She was the goddess of medicine in Ptolemaic Egypt from the third to the first centuries BC. The patient would take remedies invented by Isis which were administered along with incantations, then sleep in the temple. The cures involved plants and many other ingredients which were at times bizarre: oil, beer, wine, mother's milk, honey, resin, saliva, urine, and solid excrement. However odd these remedies, Diordorius, the Greek historian, related that Isis cured many people whom their doctors had failed.

The basis of Greek medical ethics and practices can be traced to Pharaonic Egypt. Their medical schools developed from a philosophical system and formed the prototype for later western medical practices. Hippocrates (460 to 380 BC) believed human health depended on the balance of blood, phlegm, and black and yellow bile. His greatest gift to medicine was his insistence that a physician should do no harm. Consequently, he placed emphasis on careful diagnosis and minimal intervention, often with herbal laxatives, purgatives, and emetics.

Another Greek physician, Theophrastus (370 to 285 BC), authored the *Historia Plantarum*, a classification of plants which founded the science of botany and remained the best source of herbal information until the late sixteenth century. Dioscorides' *De Materia Medica* advised on the cultivation, harvesting, medicinal preparation, and use of approximately 600 plants. Dioscorides' work, beautifully illustrated and translated into Arabic and Persian, influenced later Moslem herbals. Translated into Latin, Dioscorides' treatise, commonly known as *The Greek Herbal*, remained the most widely used physicians' textbook for several centuries.

The Romans, Pliny, Celsus and Scribonius Largus, all contributed to the medicinal knowledge of plants. Celsus' *De Medicina* mentioned more than 250 plant remedies. Galen (AD 130 to 200), a Greek surgeon at a Roman gladiatorial school before becoming a physician to the aristocracy and a pharmacist, is best known for his early contributions to our knowledge of the human circulatory, elimination, and nervous systems. Galen reported the use of cannabis both for leisure and for pain relief and prescribed extract of opium poppy for several conditions, including chronic headache, vertigo, epilepsy, asthma, colic, fevers, dropsy, leprosy, melancholy, and "troubles to which women are subject". He also won renown for his complex, often herbal concoctions which became known as galenicals.

But these medical practices were generally outside the reach of the poor. Their only hope for assistance was from the women herbalists who continued their traditional treatments in the villages. Among nomads and herders,

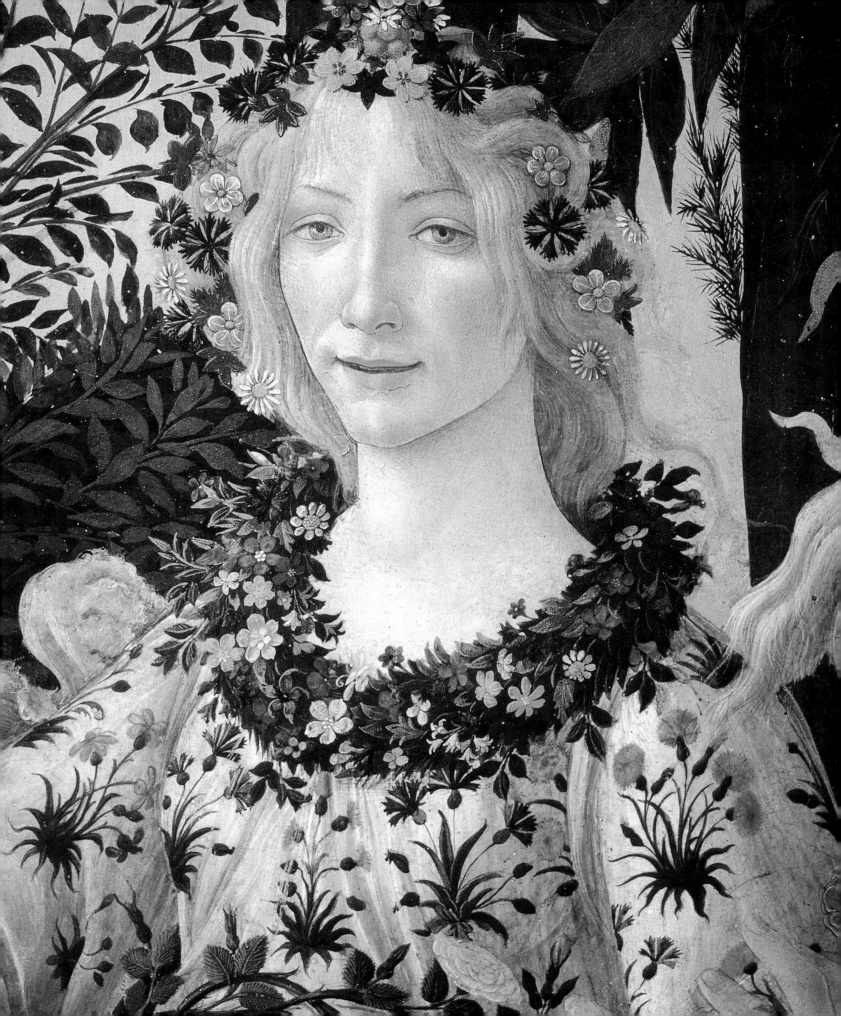

peasants, serfs, slaves, agricultural workers, and household servants, female healers were becoming known respectfully as old wives or wise-women. Their skills were learned from their mothers and grandmothers; their wisdom the cumulation of generations of experience in health and disease among their own people.

Women herbalists were both feared and respected in their communities. They were believed to possess secrets enabling them to draw on the powers of the supernatural world, a place feared as a source of evil as well as good. Though these women were generally committed to healing, at various times through history when storms, famine, plague, and other misfortunes attacked the region, the society would rise against the village wise-women in a grip of hysteria, attributing their misfortunes to the herbalist's meddling in the supernatural.

With the rise of Christianity, the situation became difficult for women herbalists. The Church began their suppression of traditional beliefs in their efforts to convert the populations of Europe by substituting pagan ceremonies with Christian ones. They competed with village healers by making churches central places of healing. In a manner similar to the practices of the Isis centuries in Egypt, the ill were encouraged to sleep in the church, and pray for heavenly intervention. The Church encouraged prayer for the cure of illness, declaring that physical disease was a sign of spiritual malaise. Rivalry sprang up between Christian magic and pagan magic. Then Theodosius I, a fourth century Roman emperor who had converted to Christianity, made paganism and all its beliefs and practices illegal. The Church regarded all magic as bad, and anyone believed to be in contact with supernatural forces was in league with the Devil. Despite this, or perhaps because of it, herbalism, superstition, magic, and Christianity in Europe following the barbarian invasions, did at times become interconnected, even among the ruling classes. Leechbooks (from the Anglo-Saxon word laece, meaning to heal) of the time contain numerous recipes for brews to ward off elves and goblins. The most famous of these was composed by a male healer, Bald, friend to Alfred the Great.

By the end of the sixth century, paganism as religion was no longer practiced, but certain rituals and beliefs were continued by individuals throughout the centuries following. As churches were the central places of healing, most medical practitioners were monks, their monastery gardens providing the raw ingredients for their medicines.

The monks preserved many Greek and Roman writings on medicine in the magnificent libraries of the great monasteries. They hand-copied these manuscripts and created extensive repositories of herbal lore. As well, they produced several treatises of their own. Odo, Bishop of Meung, described the medicinal properties of 80 plants in Latin verse in his *Viribus Herbarum*, and Batholomaeus Anglicus, an English professor of theology at Magdeburg, produced the *Liber de Proprietatibus Rerum*, an encyclopedic work including descriptions of many medicinal plants. But communities were wide spread and close knit, and women healers continued their practices within their villages.

From the twelfth century, medicine was studied in universities and became professionalized. A high degree with seven years training, medicine was practiced by lay people and was for the elite. The poor were attended by village healers, as they had been since time immemorial.

During the Christian Inquisitions which plagued the thirteenth to the eighteenth centuries, vast numbers of women healers were slain. When cures were effected and when the village flourished, the wise-women were thought to be using their powers for good. But if anything went wrong, they were accused of black magic and either arrested for trial or murdered by an enraged mob. It was claimed that as women were hostages to their senses, the female healers were more susceptible than men to satanic temptations. They were damned as the wives, daughters, and sisters of Satan, sent by him to subvert Christianity with pagan beliefs. The judgment exposed such a woman to torture designed to cleanse her immortal soul, to defeat the forces of evil which attended her, and to rescue her community from the moral danger she embodied. A barbaric public execution usually followed.

The preservation of herbal lore during the European Dark Ages owes much to the Arab empire which spread quickly east towards India and west into Spain. In Baghdad, a huge library housed an extraordinary collection of mainly Greek writings. During this period, Arab writers on medicine and pharmacy, including Rhazes (865-925) and Avicenna (930), were also active. Rhazes urged healers to prefer diet to drugs, simple remedies to complex ones. The extremely influential Avicenna's *Canon on Medicine* was outdone only by that of Ibn al-Baitar (1197-1248) of Malaga. His *Corpus of Simples* listed 1400 drugs and medicinal plants, and further developed the work of Dioscorides and Far Eastern herbals.

Following the invention of printing in the fifteenth century, hundreds of herbals were published. They were now available for the first time in English and languages other than Latin and Greek. In late sixteenth century England, William Turner produced his herbal and dedicated it to his queen, Elizabeth I. *The New Herball* is regarded as the first British Flora because it includes botanical and medicinal information on over 200 species of plants. Several sixteenth century herbals published in England and Europe were concerned with the medicinal properties of plants from the New World. John Gerard (1514-1612) discussed them extensively in *The Herball or Generall Historie Of Plantes*.

Towards the mid-seventeenth century, Charles I's herbalist, John Parkinson, published his *Theatricum Botanicum* or *Universall and Complete Herball*. This was soon outshone by Nicholas Culpeper's seminal herbal, *The English Physician Enlarged*, with "369 Medicines made of English Herbs." This blend of traditional herbal medicine, astrology, and magic was a great popular success, despite the scorn of physicians. This period also saw the introduction of active chemical drugs like arsenic, copper sulphate, iron, mercury, and sulphur.

The science of chemistry developed rapidly in the eighteenth and nineteenth centuries. Though plants were beginning to be replaced by chemicals as the primary ingredients in medicines, the first scientific treatise on the use of a folk medicine was published in the late eighteenth century. This was William Withering's *An Account of the Foxglove and Some of its Medical Uses*. In it he presented the notion that detailed assessment of individual case histories formed a sound basis of knowledge for the use of herbs.

With the immigrant settlers to America came their centuries-old home remedies. These combined with herbal wisdom learned from the Native Americans, and the tradition of American folk medicine began. Meanwhile, early nineteenth century advances in chemistry enabled the production of purer drugs from natural sources such as belladonna and hemlock, and derivatives like morphine, strychnine, atropine, and quinine; they also led to the dominance of chemical therapies which was to become the standard of the twentieth century. The nineteenth century also saw homoeopathy founded in Europe and, along with naturopathy, practiced in America.

By the turn of the twentieth century, the synthetic drug aspirin was produced. It was based on a herbal remedy and is still the largest-selling drug on the market. A wide range of the medicinal drugs commonly prescribed today originally came from plant substances or are synthetic versions of those substances.

Despite some suspicion of herbal medicine in our own times, herbalism is being continually validated by science. For instance, India's Central Drug Research Institute has investigated plants used in that continent's folk medicine. The Coleus species holds a revered place in the history of Indian herbalism. Various extracts from different types of coleus have been used since ancient Vedic times to remedy asthma, epilepsy, fever, colic, indigestion, hemorrhoids, and heart disease. Modern researchers have shown that forskolin, the main constituent of one particular coleus, affects an enzyme which counters hypertension and also increases cardiac output.

Scientists working today in some of the world's best laboratories have high hopes for their research into plants as a source of benefit to human health. Many strongly oppose the destruction of rainforests (which some estimates set at about 100 acres per minute). Rainforests are natural hothouses for thousands of plants whose medicinal value is, as yet, unknown. To destroy them is to destroy a never-to-be-repeated opportunity to add to the world's herbal-based medicine cabinet.

The popularity of medicinal plant research within the scientific community is welcomed by those millions of people concerned about the uncomfortable, and at times dangerous, side effects of some conventional medical treatments. Though modern medical schools have encouraged their graduates, and through them society, to dismiss the holistic approach to patient wellbeing emphasized by traditional herbalism, the recent and fast-growing interest in herbal medicine has made some medical practitioners aware of the efficacy of natural remedies. They are recommending these in conjunction with, or sometimes in place of, chemical drug treatments wherever they can. As well, almost every community in the western world has access to well-qualified herbalists and natural healers.

Herbalism survives and prospers, its emphasis on a healer's sympathy with the trials of the human condition now recognized as essentially good medicine.

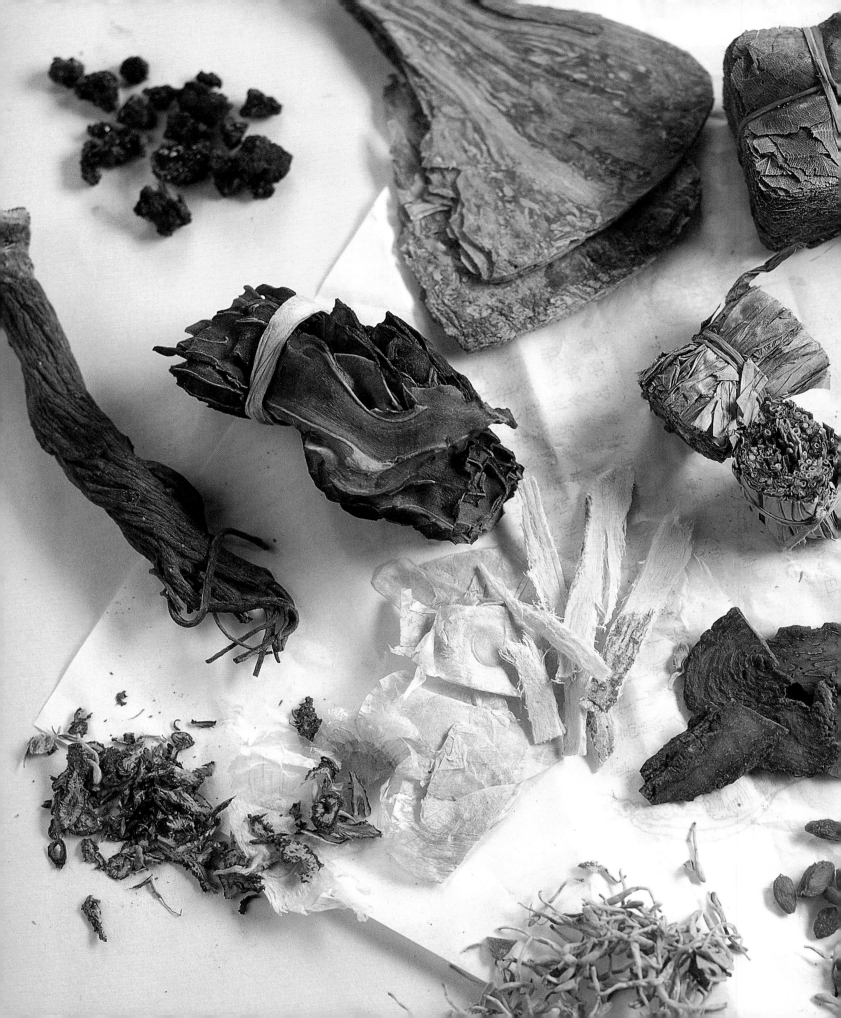

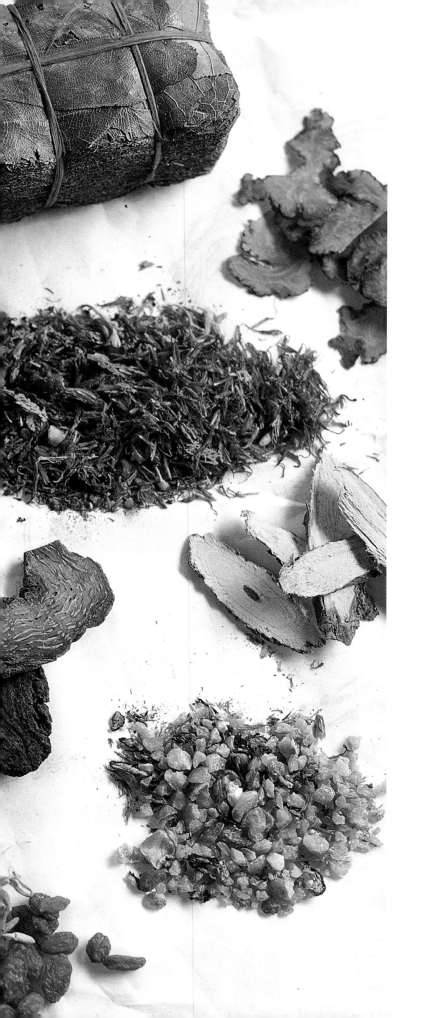

Chinese Herbal Medicine

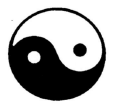

The practice of Chinese herbalism is a very particular and highly complex skill. Qualified practitioners, however, can be found world-wide, and this form of herbalism continues to grow in popularity in countries outside of China, along with other forms of Chinese Medicine.

Traditional Chinese medicine is a total health care and maintenance system. It includes internal medicine (Chinese herbal, animal and mineral remedies), Qi Gong (Chinese breathing exercises), Tai Qi Chuan (physical exercises), Tuina (Chinese massage), bone setting, acupuncture, and Chinese dietary therapy.

These various practices are based on a central philosophy which owes much to the early Taoist philosophers who taught the importance of balance in life.

The fundamental principle of traditional Chinese medicine is to establish and maintain by regular review and adjustment, the body's ideal internal balance which promotes health and longevity.

Ch'i (or Qi) refers to the lifeforce of the body. This energy flows through channels in the body in much the same way as blood flows through veins and arteries. These channels are called meridians. Each corresponds to a particular body organ and its energy flow corresponds to fluctuations in the body's electromagnetic field. The meridians, although separate channels, do overlap the circulatory and the central nervous systems.

Ch'i energy is composed of the counter-balancing elements of Yin and Yang. In the poetic Chinese manner, Yin is described as the shady side of the mountain, Yang the sunny side. Yin is understood as passive, cold, contracting, internal, negative, and feminine. By contrast, Yang is active, warm, expanding, external, positive, and masculine. The terms "positive" and "negative" are not value judgments but indicate polarity.

Both Yin and Yang elements are always present in the body and in constant flux. If an imbalance lasts too long or is too severe, illness will result. For instance, too much Yin may cause a chill, too much Yang a fever. If you are too Yin, you might be lethargic, feel the cold, catch cold easily, perhaps be pale or even anaemic. If you are too Yang, you might be hot-tempered, your pulse excessively fast or strong, your skin reddish or prone to rash.

Poetic symbolism is also used to describe the distinct roles of the body's organs. The body is compared to an Empire, the heart to an Emperor or Overlord, the key organs to ministers of state. The lungs are cast as the Prime Minister, the kidneys as Minister for Health, the gall bladder as Minister for Justice, the liver as the alert General responsible for protective strategies and communications.

As all decisions by the ministers should be referred to the Emperor, the heart, then, is the ultimate authority. The mind, as the seat of being, comes within the realm of the heart, the Emperor, and is treated separately to the brain.

The Chinese characterize the body's organs by observing the relationship between each organ and various emotions. For example, to express anger — or liver energy — without referring your response to the Emperor heart, indicates some imbalance in the flow of energy from liver to heart which could trigger a chain of imbalance in other parts of the body.

The organs are also associated with the elements: heart with fire, spleen with earth, lungs with air (sometimes called metal), kidneys with water, and liver with wood. The liver is associated with wood because the ancient Chinese realized, long before Western medical practitioners, that the liver is the only organ capable of tissue regeneration as is the wood of living trees. The poetic image of the organs as natural elements is also used to describe the ideal flow of energy throughout the body: fire from the sun energizes the earth to create vegetation which in turn affects the air which compounds to metal. Air/metal condenses to water which gives life to trees/wood which burns to create fire. And so the cycle continues.

The Chinese also categorize each organ as primarily Yin or Yang. Yin characterizes lungs, spleen, heart, pericardium, kidneys, and liver. Yang dominates the large intestine, stomach, small intestine, bladder, and gall bladder.

Although many Western-educated doctors are interested in the entire field of Chinese medicine, most accept at least some parts of the Chinese system. Some forms, like acupuncture, have been more readily taken up than others. In the realm of herbalism, tastebuds familiar only with Western food often need time to adjust to Chinese herbal soups, which can be unusually powerful in taste, and should be sipped, not swallowed in one gulp.

Indeed, the slow and steady approach is intrinsic to Chinese herbalism which, like the herbalism of the West, does not pursue overnight cures. If yours is a chronic condition, a few courses of herbal treatment are usually necessary to restore your internal balance of Yin and Yang and the healthy flow of Ch'i.

*The Chinese herbalist uses the
12 pulses (six in each wrist) to help their
diagnosis. The pulses give the herbalist
insight into the balance of Yin and Yang in
the body. They will also check the tongue
and the skin, eyes and hair.*

Using Chinese herbs

Dried and granulated Chinese herbs and herbal teas, all of which promote healthy living and are acceptable to the novice Western palate, are available over the counter. If you have a serious or obstinate condition, you will need to see a qualified Chinese herbalist for a correct diagnosis and herbal remedy designed for your specific needs.

Temperature control

Chinese herbalists believe you must protect your internal Yin-Yang balance against external destabilizers such as heat, cold, wind, and damp. Their advice is that in cool weather you keep neck, shoulders, and lower back area warm. If you have painful knees, ankles, or other joints, keep them warm too. In hot weather, take care not to overexert yourself, dehydrate, or get sunburnt. Chinese herbalists also advise a diet of one-third cold food to two-thirds hot, except in very hot weather. They maintain that a greater proportion of cold foods encourages excessive Yin by chilling the stomach, impairing the function of certain organs, and lowering energy levels. They caution against unlimited quantities of refrigerated foods such as raw salad vegetables or fruit, icecream, or iced water. Similarly, overly hot or spicy foods can have a detrimental effect if your energy levels tend to be too Yang or hot.

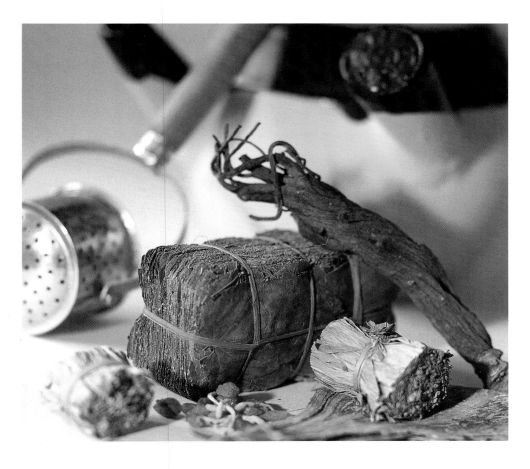

*The herbalist will prescribe
a selection of herbs in various combinations which
can then be simmered with water in
a Chinese soup pot until reduced and then drunk.*

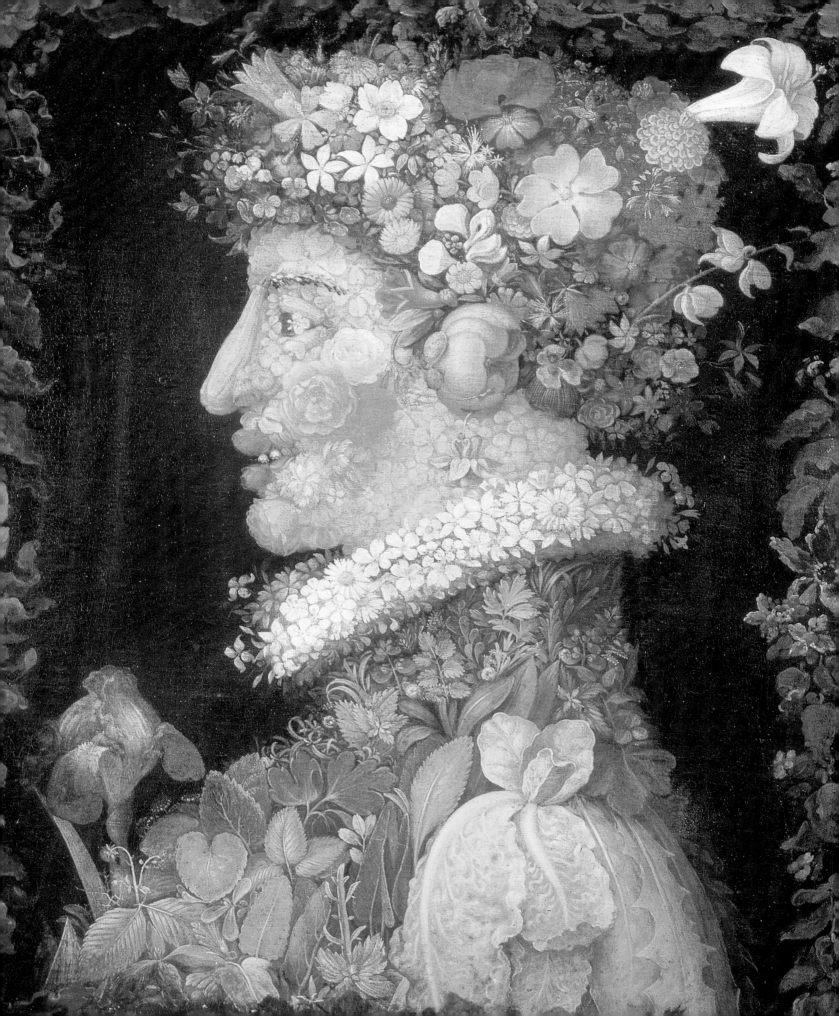

Bach Flower Remedies

Although these remedies are chosen in line with psychological states, they can also be used to treat physical ailments — often linked to emotions — as they are designed to treat the whole person and their internal imbalance, not just an illness.

In the 1930s, the British doctor Edward Bach formulated his Bach Flower Remedies, herbal medications to assist in healing the conflict between spirit and ego which he saw as fundamental to ill health.

Early in his distinguished, orthodox medical career, Dr Bach decided that the best method of medical education was the observation of patients' reactions to disease, and that the main fault of modern medical science was to treat effects rather than causes.

In the course of practicing at London's University College Hospital and at his private consultation rooms in Harley Street, Dr Bach became dissatisfied with the success rate of orthodox medicine, noting that patients who enjoyed permanent recovery were rare while others made only scant improvement or suffered relapses.

He began to search for more efficacious treatment, a quest which led him to explore many fields of medical research. He won acclaim for his work on vaccines as Assistant Bacteriologist at the University College Hospital and during the First World War when his responsibilities included a huge war casualty ward.

In July 1917, Dr Bach was given three months to live and he determined to complete his current research before his death. He noticed that far from declining quickly under this stress, his health improved. His experience led him to conclude that a sense of purpose in life was fundamental to good health.

Following his recovery, he continued to practice orthodox medicine, gaining further professional distinction during the influenza epidemic of 1918 when his vaccines saved the lives of thousands.

Soon after, he read *The Organon of the Healing Art* by Samuel Hahnemann, the founder of homoeopathy. Hahnemann's philosophy was to treat the sufferer, not the illness, and he obtained most of his remedies from animal, vegetable, and mineral matter.

Dr Bach next joined the London Homoeopathic Hospital while continuing to manage his increasingly popular private practice. He defined what he called the Seven Nosodes, oral vaccines that worked on organisms present in the intestines. He also advocated a diet of uncooked fruits, vegetables, cereals, and nuts to reduce toxins in the intestines.

Bach Flower Remedies,
available from health food stores,
herbalists, and naturopaths,
are taken by placing drops
beneath the tongue.

In 1928, Dr Bach hypothesized that people could be categorized as personality types whose similar responses to a variety of illnesses presented a useful frame of reference for diagnosis and treatment.

This theory, his supposition that if distress could affect one's appearance it might also adversely effect internal bodily organs, and his study of Hahnemann, encouraged Dr Bach to abandon his London-based work. He would investigate the effects of simple, herbal medicines on human thoughts and feelings, and anticipated that the sources of these remedies would be found in the countryside.

From 1930 until his death in 1936, Bach walked Wales and England, observing nature and developing the Bach Flower Remedies. During this time, he discovered that his sensitivity to plants increased so that he could hold a flower and feel the effects of the bloom's properties in his body. Sometimes a flower would leave him feeling uplifted, at other times nauseous or faint.

Dr Bach focused on flowers because he believed the essence of a plant was concentrated in its flower before seeding. He extracted the essence by placing picked flowerheads in a bowl of water left in the sun for several hours to receive solar energization before being stabilized with brandy.

Dr Bach listed 38 plants with healing properties, including the twelve plants he listed in *The Twelve Healers and Other Remedies*. His remedies can be used singly or in combination, and Dr Bach urged their use in conjunction with other forms of treatment. Recent decades have witnessed renewed interest in Dr Bach's healing philosophy and his Flower Remedies which seem to be devoid of side effects. One of the best known is Rescue Remedy, a composite herbal liquid used to treat shock or distress. It can be particularly helpful to children and animals, calming them almost instantly.

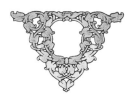

Unhealthy moods and personality types and their Bach Flower Remedies

Mostly unhappy — *Holly*
Panicky — *Rock Rose*
Fear of losing control — *Cherry Plum*
Absorbed by memories — *Honeysuckle*
Self-absorption — *Heather*
Desire to be alone — *Water Violet*
Dislike of being alone — *Chicory, Heather*
Unambitious — *Clematis, Gorse, Wild Rose*
Anxious — *Agrimony*
Sulky — *Willow*
Strict with others — *Beech, Vine*
Vexatious — *Holly, Pine*
Talkative — *Honeysuckle, Vervain*
Apathetic — *Clematis, Wild Rose*
Worry over other's troubles — *Red Chestnut*
Drains others' vitality — *Vervain, Cerato, Vine*
Not clear about ambitions — *Oat*
Feeling suicidal — *Aspen, Cherry Plumb, Mimulus*
A struggler — *Oat*
Tearful — *Scleranthus*
Self pity — *Heather, Willow*
Gives in to setbacks — *Gorse*
Sensitive to noise — *Clematis, Mimulus*

There are many more moods and remedies to counter them. If you are in doubt about which remedy to take, consult an expert.

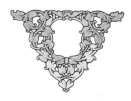

The 38 Bach Flower Remedies and conditions treated

Agrimony
Mental torture; worry, concealed from others

Aspen
Vague fears of unknown origin; anxiety; apprehension

Beech
Intolerance; criticism; passing judgements

Centaury
Weak willed; too easily influenced; willing servitors

Cerato
Distrust of self; doubt of one's ability; foolishness

Cherry Plum
Desperation; fear of losing control of the mind;
dread of doing some frightful thing

Chestnut Bud
Failure to learn by experience; lack of observation in the
lessons of life — hence the need of repetition

Chicory
Possessiveness; self-love; self-pity

Clematis
Indifference; dreaminess; inattention; unconsciousness

Crab Apple
The cleansing remedy; despondency; despair

Elm
Occasional feelings of inadequacy; despondency;
exhaustion from over-striving for perfection

Gentian
Doubt; depression; discouragement

Gorse
Hopelessness: despair

Heather
Self-centeredness; self-concern

Holly
Hatred; envy; jealousy; suspicion

Honeysuckle
Dwelling upon thoughts of the past; nostalgia;
homesickness

Hornbeam
Tiredness; weariness; mental and physical exhaustion

Impatiens
Impatience; irritability; extreme mental tension

Larch
Lack of confidence; anticipation of failure;despondency

Mimulus
Fear or anxiety of a known origin

Oak
Despondency; despair — but ceaseless effort

Olive
Complete exhaustion; mental fatigue

Pine
Self-reproach; guilt feelings; despondency

Red Chestnut
Excessive fear; anxiety for others

Rock Rose
Terror; panic; extreme fright

Rock water
Self-repression; self-denial; self-martyrdom

Scleranthus
Uncertainty; indecision; hesitancy; imbalance

Star of Bethlehem
Shock, mental or physical

Sweet Chestnut
Extreme mental anguish; hopelessness; despair

Vervain
Strain; stress; tension; over-enthusiasm

Vine
Dominating; inflexible; ambitious

Walnut
Over-sensitive to ideas and influences

Water Violet
Pride; aloofness

White Chestnut
Persistent unwanted thoughts; mental arguments
and conversations

Wild Oat
Uncertainty; despondency; dissatisfaction

Wild Rose
Resignation; apathy

Willow
Resentment; bitterness

Rescue Remedy comprises:
Star of Bethlehem for shock
Rock Rose for terror and panic
Impatiens for mental stress and tension
Cherry Plum for desperation
Clematis for the disassociation which can precede fainting
or unconsciousness

A Herbal Selection

*This chapter provides an easy-to-follow guide
to some of the most commonly used herbs — plants that you can grow
in your own garden and herbal treatments you can use at home.*

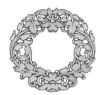

ALOE
Aloe vera

Part used: fleshy leaves

History and mythology
Aloe vera is commonly known as "medicinal plant",
a reference to the healing quality of the thick, clear liquid
stored in its leaves. The ancient Greeks and Romans as
well as the Arabians, Indians, and Chinese relied on aloe
and the famous Ebers Papyrus (1500 BC) chronicles its
widespread use. Cleopatra is said to have used the gel as a
beauty cream.

Harvesting and processing
Cut leafblades, squeeze out thick juice and apply
immediately to affected area. It is not safe to store this
juice for more than one to two days, even when
refrigerated. A weak solution for internal use can be stored
under refrigeration for one week. Mix approximately two
teaspoons of leaf peelings per cup of water. Preserved aloe
vera liquid and aloe tablets can be purchased commercially.

Medicinal use
Apply the gel directly to skin to heal burns, blemishes,
wounds, and skin irritations. The fresh gel can be consumed
daily as a tonic to aid kidney infections, as a mild laxative,
to expel worms, and to assist arthritis and ulcers. In tablet
form, aloe vera treats digestive complaints.

ANGELICA
Angelica archangelica

Part used: leaves, roots, seeds, stalks

History and mythology
The lore of northern Europe, especially of Lapland,
Iceland, and Russia, often mentions angelica. According to
one legend, Michael the Archangel revealed to a monk in
the Middle Ages that the plant would cure the plague.
Thus the origin of its Latin name: *angelica archangelica*.
Angelica was certainly used to fight the plague and often
featured in monastery gardens.

Harvesting and processing
Angelica's essential oil content is intensified by up to
80 per cent if the common stinging nettle, *Urtica dioica*,
is planted as its companion. To harvest good quality leaves
and stems, remove the flowering heads as soon as they
appear. Harvest the seed just before it starts to fall,
by snipping off and drying whole flowerheads. Harvest
the leaves by separating from the stems. Wash and store
angelica root in a dry, well-ventilated place until needed.

Medicinal use
Since one of angelica's constituents is the digestive enzyme
pectin, chewing slowly on its stalks is recommended for
flatulence or other digestive discomfort. Tea made from
any of its parts warms the body, promotes sweating and
eases rheumatism. It soothes nerves and relieves colds and
flu, sore throats, coughs, and bronchitis. It is also reputed to
produce aversion to alcohol. In Chinese herbalism, the root
(*dang gui*) of *angelica sinensis*, is used to make a powerful
general tonic. (Diabetics are warned to avoid angelica as it
may destabilize blood sugar levels.)

SWEET BASIL
Ocimum basilicum

Part used: leaves

History and mythology
Basil originated in India, where it was regarded as a sacred herb. It was also known in ancient Egypt, Greece, and Rome. Its name might come from the Greek *basileus* (king) to suggest the plant's sovereign or highly efficacious healing quality. Or it might refer to the plant's historic association with the basilisk, a mythical, serpentine creature with a crown-like crest and fiery, death-dealing eyes. The seventeenth century herbalist Jacques Tournefourt was convinced that enhaling the scent of basil would cause scorpions to breed in one's brain, and for many years the plant was linked with poison although basil poultices were prescribed to draw poison from stings and bites.

Harvesting and processing
In hot climates, basil grows and may be harvested fresh as needed throughout the year. In cold climates, dry the remains of the late summer crop of outdoor plants before the first frost. Fresh basil leaves may be chopped finely, mixed with water and frozen as icecubes. In the garden, basil and rue are hostile plantings.

Medicinal use
Basil is recommended as a remedy for diseases of the brain, heart, lungs, kidneys, and bladder. It is often mixed with borage to make a tonic tea to revive lowered vitality. Essential oil of basil as a bath or massage oil has a relaxing effect. A snuff of dried basil leaves or an inhalation made by pouring boiling water over fresh leaves may relieve colds and headaches, nervousness, nervous stomach disorders, and insomnia. Leaves applied directly to the skin give relief from insect bites and itching.

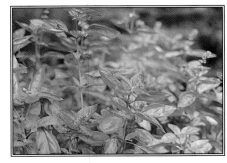
Sweet Basil

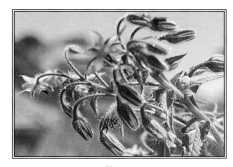
Borage

BORAGE
Borago officinalis

Part used: flowers, leaves, seeds

History and mythology
Borage, native to the Mediterranean, travelled with the Romans throughout Europe and into Asia and from there to the Middle East. Early European migrants to the New World carried it with them to North America. Its flowers are emblematic of bravery and borage tea was drunk to engender courage. One school of thought traces its name to the old Celtic *borrach* meaning courage, another to the Latin *cor ago* for "I stimulate the heart", while its Arabic name *abourach* translates as "father of sweat". All these names make a lot of sense when one discovers that modern research has shown that the herb stimulates adrenalin production. Borage can assist the treatment of stress, depression, grief, or anxiety.

Harvesting and processing
Borage leaves and flowers may be used fresh in any season. Before drying, separate the flowers, leaves, and stalks.

Medicinal use
Borage is rich in potassium, calcium, mineral acids, and a very beneficial saline mucilage. Its dried and crushed leaves were used to cleanse the blood and assist circulation. The urinary tract is said to respond well to a borage infusion which also induces sweating to hasten the healing of fevers, chills, measles, influenza, and the common cold. Borage leaf compresses help relieve congested veins, especially those in the legs caused by lengthy standing. Oil from the seeds is used in capsule form to treat rheumatic and menstrual disorders, and eczema. Borage is related to another healing herb, comfrey, and blends well with basil in herbal tea.

CAYENNE
Capsicum frutescens minimum

Part used: fruits

History and mythology
These plants were grown by the Inca people of South America. Christopher Columbus probably found them in Cuba and introduced them to Europe, although it is also possible that cayenne first arrived in England from India in the mid-sixteenth century.

Harvesting and processing
Pick when ripe and dry whole before grinding pods and seeds together to produce a light orange to red, coarse-textured powder.

Medicinal use
Cayenne is a potent stimulant for the whole body as well as having antiseptic and antibacterial properties. It warms the body and promotes sweating. It is thus used to stimulate the digestion and the circulation and is excellent for chills, colds, flu, and respiratory ailments as well as all manner of throat problems. Try a little blended with a mixture of cucumber, onions, lime juice, and madeira, as it may assist weak digestion and loss of appetite. Tea made with approximately one-eighth of a teaspoon of cayenne powder per cup of water can be taken three times daily, or the same amount of cayenne may be added to other hot drinks. The same tea added to a little more warm water makes an excellent hand or footbath for people who suffer from poor circulation or winter chilblains. Compresses or a massage oil can be used for rheumatism, arthritis, sprains, and bruising. Because it is a very hot spice, use with great caution when preparing, handling, and using.

Gentle but effective chamomile is one of the easiest herbs to incorporate into everyday life, and also one of the most popular in commercial preparations.

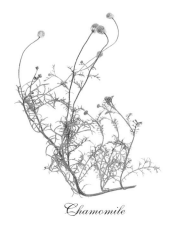
Chamomile

CHAMOMILE
Matricaria chamomilla or recutita (German)
Anthemis nobile (Roman)

Part used: flowers

History and mythology
The Egyptian priests were aware of chamomile's curative powers (as were the ancient Greeks and Romans) and dedicated it to Ra, their sun god. India's Ayurvedic physicians used it to relieve digestive complaints, cramps, and fever. The early Vikings used chamomile rinses to enhance their blondness. The Anglo Saxons called it maythen and deemed it sacred. The Spaniards called it manzanilla, meaning 'little apple'. In Britain, chamomile has been used for centuries as an insect repellent, and in pleasant, comforting baths for healthy and sick alike.

Harvesting
One of chamomile's folk names is "plant physician" as it is widely beneficial in the garden. The prized chamomile flowers should be harvested early in the day before the sun draws the valuable, volatile essences from the blossoms.

Medicinal use
Chamomile tea is famous as a mild sedative to promote calm sleep, soothe frayed nerves, disturbed digestion, and premenstrual symptoms. Tired or restless children also benefit from a mild chamomile tea which is also suitable for all sufferers of colds and fevers. An infusion of the flowers, strained and poured into a hot bath, will reduce muscular weariness and fatigue. A well-tried folk remedy for eye problems is frequent bathing with strained, cooled, chamomile tea. A sachet of warm, dry chamomile is said to soothe earache and neuralgia. Topically, the herb reduces skin irritations. A sachet steeped in hot but tolerable water is recommended to soothe facial swellings.

CHICKWEED
Stellaria media

Part used: leaves, stems

History and mythology
In many languages, this herb is associated with birds. In French it is *herbe a l'oiseau*; in German *vogelmiere*; in Latin *morsus gallinae* or hen's bite. In winter, it is often one of the few sources of fresh, nutritious seed for wild birds, while in summer they benefit from the high iron and copper content of its foliage.

Harvesting and processing
Because chickweed flowers only briefly, prepare to harvest it at the first appearance of its small white flowers. Cut the stalks close to the ground, remove the flowerheads, and gather the stalks and leaves into loose bundles to hang or spread thinly to dry.

Medicinal use
Chickweed is a good, easily consumable source of iron and copper, and thus can prove valuable in the diets of menstruating women and girls who pursue an athletic lifestyle. It is also a natural diuretic and eases the discomfort of fluid retention. An infusion of chickweed is a soothing eyebath and, with the addition of lemon juice and honey, can be drunk to ease constipation. Its leaves can be used in a poultice to relieve rheumatic and arthritic discomfort, the itching and irritation of eczema and other skin rashes, and to heal persistent ulcers. Made into an ointment, it is said to cure chilblains. Added to a bath, it will generally sooth and heal sunburned or otherwise tender skin over large surfaces of the body. A drawing poultice of slippery elm powder and chickweed is effective on boils.

CHILI
Capsicum frutescens annuum

Part used: fruit

History and mythology
The Chinese claim that the chili is indigenous to their Szechuan region and chilies were certainly cultivated at least 9000 years ago in Mexico which is their more probable country of origin. From Mexico they spread north to become part of the herbal history of the American Indians. To the south, they reached Venezuela whose migratory Arawak and Carib tribes introduced them to the West Indies. In 1492, Columbus came across them in Hispaniola and by the sixteenth century there were plantings in Spain and Portugal. From here the chili travelled to Japan and India to become one of that continent's most important spices. From India it was taken to Arabia along the old spice routes.

Harvesting and processing
In both garden and kitchen, whole fresh chilies must be handled with care, preferably with gloves, or they may do you more harm than good. Use a small, sharp, pointed knife to slice them in half lengthways and to scrape out and discard the seeds. If not wearing gloves, be wary of rubbing your eyes or face or licking your fingers when handling them. Chili powder, less hot and more flavorsome than cayenne pepper, is actually a mixture of dried and ground chilies, ground cumin, oregano, and garlic.

Medicinal use
As well as being a warming stimulant that promotes sweating, we now know that fresh chilies are a rich source of vitamin C, a fact that adds weight to the traditional use of an infusion of dried or ground chilies to treat chills and fever. Chilies may also be added to creams or ointments to warm and massage sore, aching muscles. In India, the chili is used to stimulate the appetite of convalescents.

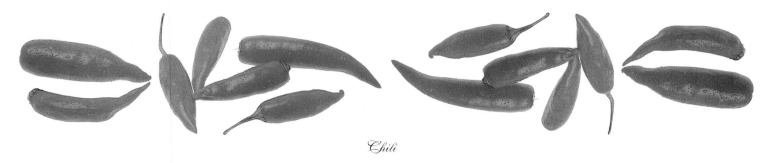

Chili

COMFREY
Symphytum officinale

Part used: leaves, roots

History and mythology
Comfrey's names are derived from the Greek *sympho* to unite and the Latin *confervere* meaning "to grow together." It enjoys many folk names including boneset, knitbone, and bruisewort in reference to the healing powers appreciated by country folk for centuries.

Harvesting and processing
Comfrey leaves and roots are more effective fresh but can be useful when dried in the ordinary way.

Medicinal use
The pureed leaves and a paste from the powdered comfrey root can be applied as a poultice to ease sprains and bruises, staunch clean but bleeding wounds, and heal minor fractures. Oil infusions can be used for arthritis. Its main healing element is its constituent allantoin, which encourages cell growth in muscles, bones, and cartilage. There has been some debate about the toxicity of comfrey when taken internally, but a weak infusion of leaves or roots has remedied stomach ulcers, coughs and chest colds, circulatory problems and intestinal distress. Added to bathwater, it soothes tender skin and eases eczema.

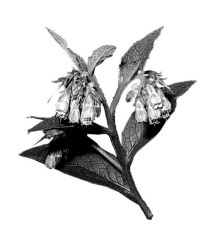

Comfrey

Professional herbalists often prescribe echinacea in commercial formulations to treat all manner of illness, as these can provide an effective alternative to modern pharmaceuticals.

ECHINACEA
Echinacea angustifolia

History and mythology
Echinacea was fundamental to the medicine kit of the indigenous tribes who inhabited the plains of North America. They used the roots for poultices to treat wounds, snakebite, and insect bites and stings. They made infusions to rinse painful teeth and gums and a drink to treat colds, arthritis, and later, the smallpox and measles introduced by Europeans.

Harvesting and processing
The black roots of this herb should be three to four years old before harvesting. Then, after the plant has flowered, the roots can be washed, chopped and dried.

Medicinal use
Echinacea is renowned for its effectiveness against infections be they viral, fungal, or bacterial. It both attacks the harmful invaders and assists the body's own immune system. It is used to relieve acute infections, for example: colds and sore throats, abscesses or skin eruptions, oral or vaginal thrush, and urinary tract infections. Longer term problems such as chronic bronchitis, sinusitis, or female pelvic infections may also respond to echinacea. It may be prescribed for internal use as a tea to be taken three times daily, or as a mouthwash, douche, or decoction.

ELDER
Sambucus nigra

Part used: bark, berries, flowers, leaves

History and mythology
The elder grows wild in many parts of Europe and belongs to the folklore of a number of countries. The Anglo-Saxons called it Eldrun. Danish legend connected it with magic, believing that in the branches dwelt a dryad, Hylde-Moer, the Elder Tree Mother, and that if one stood under the tree on Midsummer Eve one would see the King of Fairyland and all his train ride by. Russian peasants said that the compassionate spirit of the elder would drive away evil and also give long life. The Sicilians thought that sticks made of its wood killed serpents and drove away robbers, and the English folk believed that the elder was never struck by lightning.

Harvesting and processing
As elder trees have a long flowering period from summer to autumn, harvesting them for drying and storing may be an ongoing, leisurely task. Gather the flowers when the buds are open and before midday so as not to lose too much of the floral essence. Leave some flowers on the trees for fresh use to ensure the later development of berries. The shiny green berries, to be used fresh or when dried, first appear in autumn and should be picked as they turn reddish purple.

Medicinal use
Once described as "the medicine chest of the country people", *Sambucus nigra* possesses more therapeutic qualities than any other species of elder and all its parts are useful. Hippocrates used elder bark as a purgative and the green inner bark makes a soothing, all-purpose lubricant ointment. Ointment made from the flowers heals burns and chilblains. The leaves are also used in ointments, and as a wash, to repair and soothe the skin. Elder root tea was considered the best remedy for dropsy, and a strained infusion of fresh or dried elderflowers alleviates inflamed eyes. Elderflower tea — peppermint leaves optional — promotes perspiration and is an old influenza remedy; it soothes inflamed nasal passages and relieves sinusitis and catarrh. Elderberry wine, mildly laxative and diuretic, relieves sciatic, rheumatic, and arthritic pain. Elderberry juice was used as a laxative and for colic.
A cooled infusion of bitter elder leaves dabbed on the face is advised to repel insects such as mosquitoes and flies.

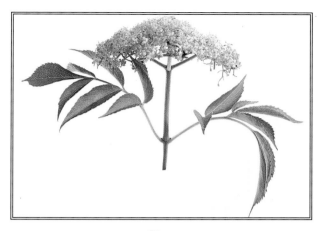
Elder

GARLIC
Allium sativum

Part used: corm

History and mythology
Homer, Pliny, Virgil, Horace, Chaucer, and Shakespeare wrote about garlic which was an important part of the Egyptian, Roman, and Greek diets. The people who worked to build the Pyramids consumed garlic as a ritual and to promote good health. The Greek physician Galen described is as the people's *thereac* or cure-all.

Harvesting and processing
Harvesting usually takes place about six months after planting, when the flowers are fading and leaves are yellowing. The bulbs are hung in a dry atmosphere to avoid mildew until hardened, when they should be stored in a ventilated container in a cool, dry place.

Medicinal use
Garlic has remarkable medicinal properties and is a powerful antiseptic. It contains the vitamins A, B, and C, as well as copper, sulphur, manganese, iron, and calcium. When a garlic clove is crushed, a natural chemical interaction triggers the plant's antiseptic potential (it targets only harmful bacteria) as well as its distinctive odor. Eating crushed garlic is recommended to soothe infected digestive systems, and as it is absorbed into the bloodstream, it continues its good work throughout the body on upper and lower respiratory tract infections and in controlling fat deposits, the cause of hardened arteries, angina, and high blood pressure. Garlic capsules are available, but keep in mind that deodorized preparations are less effective as the active constituents are altered when removing odor. Chewing sprigs of fresh parsley may freshen the breath.

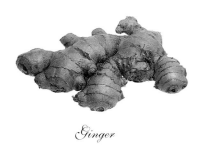

Ginger

GINGER
Zingiber officinale

Part used: rhizome (root)

History and mythology
Ginger now grows all over the world but is indigenous to south-east Asia, first arriving in Europe about 2000 BC. Traditional Chinese Medicine uses the fresh root (*sheng jiang*), the peeled root skin (*jiang pi*) and the dried root (*gan jiang*), the latter being seen as an effective Yang restorative. It is used to reduce the toxicity of other herbs, and in the eighteenth century was added to remedies to modify possible irritative reactions.

Harvesting and processing
A ginger plant should not be harvested until at least one year old. Then, after the flowers and leaves have died down, the rhizome is retrieved from the soil. To store fresh, green ginger, slice finely or mince and cover with sherry in a sterilized, airtight container, or scald it, soak in water for three days — changing the water daily — then peel before steeping in a strong mixture of boiled water and sugar syrup. To dry the rhizome, first scrape, then wash (but do not scald because this reduces the flavor) before leaving to dry thoroughly in a cool, airy place.

Medicinal use
Ginger has a long history as a remedy for flatulence and indigestion along with other herbs and spices such as tansy, fennel, dill, rosemary, anise, the mints, cardamom, nutmeg, cloves, and cinnamon. In Indian Ayurvedic medicine, ginger is used as a carminative and to remedy dyspepsia. It is used in all forms of herbalism for its warming and stimulating properties: to dispel chills, promote sweating, and boost circulation. It can help stop vomiting, diarrhea, and bleeding, and has antispasmodic and antiseptic qualities. As candied ginger or ginger pills, the herb is also effective in preventing motion sickness. A tea made with freshly grated ginger relieves cold symptoms and coughs.

HYSSOP
Hyssopus officinalis

Part used: flowers, leaves, and sometimes stems

History and mythology
Hyssop is native to southern Europe, and was well known in the ancient world. Its early recorded name *azob*, a holy herb, referred to its use for purification rites in Egyptian temples. The conquering Romans are said to have introduced hyssop wherever they went, valuing it as both a ceremonial and healing plant. Monastery gardens were planted with hyssop for religious and medicinal purposes.

Harvesting and processing
Dried hyssop flowers are used extensively in herbal medicine, and are harvested during peak blossoming time in late summer. The leaves may be harvested at any time.

Medicinal use
Hyssop has expectorant, carminative, and antispasmodic qualities, and helps promote sweating, making it an important ingredient in many chest, appetite, digestive, and gastric tonics and in herbal treatments to aid urine excretion, to expel worms, and to soothe a sore throat. Hyssop flower tea will help relieve a heavy cold or digestive disorders. Hyssop foliage tea taken several times daily is a folk cure for rheumatism and is an antiseptic, healing bath for cuts and bruises. Topically, hyssop has anti-inflammatory properties.

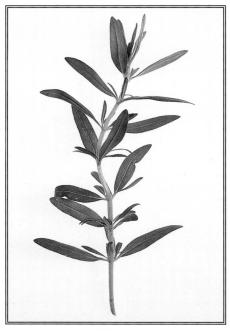

Hyssop

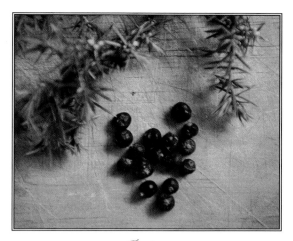
Juniper

JUNIPER
Juniperus communus

Part used: ripe berries, leaves

History and mythology
In the Middle Ages, a juniper bush planted by the door of a house was said to keep witches away, juniper branches were burned to prevent plague and in World War II, French nurses burned juniper to disinfect the air in field hospitals. Nicolas Culpeper recognized juniper was a diuretic and also prescribed it for "cough, shortness of breath," and "to give safe and speedy delivery to women with child". The ancient Egyptians used juniper oil in the embalming process.

Harvesting and processing
The juniper berry's essential oil is extracted at its peak just before the ripening and darkening of the fruit. The leafy branchlets also contain many of the same substances. Juniper berries may be used fresh or when dried.

Medicinal use
The medicinal properties of juniper berry tea relieve flatulence, help release fluid in kidneys and bladder, ease menstrual symptoms, alleviate gout, chest complaints, rheumatism, and arthritis. The herb stimulates blood circulation, aids resistance to internal infections, alleviates urinary infections, and is an appetite and digestion enhancer. Externally, juniper oil diluted with olive oil helps relieve aching joints and certain skin disorders. Some herbalists recommend juniper oil as an inhalant for bronchitis, or as a chest rub for a cough. Do not use juniper when kidneys or bladder are inflamed, or during pregnancy.

Herbal Essential Oils

The active ingredients in plants are known as essential oils. These pure, concentrated essences can be extracted and then used for their fragrance and their therapeutic value. The oils can be used in vaporizers, atomizers, baths, light bulb rings, in massage oils, and cosmetic preparations. This is known as the practice of aromatherapy. Essential oils can be used as an adjunct to other herbal treatments. Some popular herbs and herbal flowers from which essential oils are extracted are basil, bergamot, chamomile, fennel, geranium, lavender, lemongrass, peppermint, rose, rosemary, and thyme. These herbal essential oils have therapeutic properties that work not only towards alleviating physical ailments and health conditions but also on a psychological and emotional level. The sense of smell is one of the most direct triggers of our emotions and the proper use of essential oils can calm the nerves, dispel fears, and uplift the spirits from despondency. For instance, essential oil of lavender is calming and relaxing, and essential oil of rosemary is stimulating and refreshing. Purchase oils from a reputable supplier, and do not confuse them with cheaper aromatic or fragrant oils which do not contain the essential active ingredients.

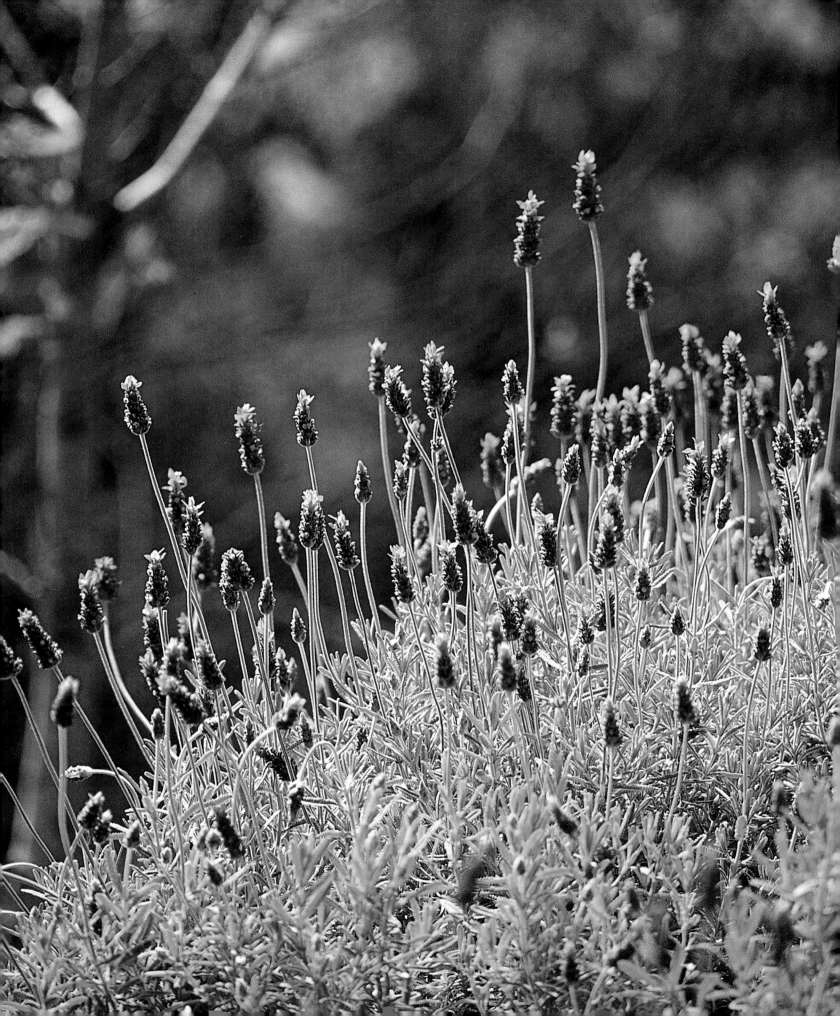

LAVENDER
Lavandula augustifolia
Lavandula spica
Lavandula officinalis

Part used: flowers, leaves

History and mythology
All of the many types of lavender are native to the Mediterranean countries, although only some are used medicinally. English lavender, cultivated in Britain from the late sixteenth century, was originally used by the ancient Greeks. The Arabs used lavender as an expectorant and antispasmodic, and the Europeans found it healed wounds and expelled worms. From Elizabethan times, oil of lavender has protected stored linens against moths and silverfish — rubbed over doors and furniture, it deters lice, fleas, and flies.

Harvesting and processing
Lavender is best picked when its oil content is highest, that is, before the last flowers on each stalk are fully opened and early on a dry day, before the sun absorbs the volatile essence. Bunch and hang, blooms downwards, in a cool, airy place until dry. Flowers will then strip easily from the stalks for storage.

Medicinal use
Lavender is a delightfully fragrant reviver for anyone feeling jangled or stressed. Although an infusion of the flowers can be used and makes a useful sedative tea, it is the essential oil of lavender which is far more potent. A bath at night with a few drops of the oil soothes and relaxes the peripheral nerves. Lavender counters giddiness and faintness, nervous palpitations, flatulence, indigestion and the discomfort of rheumatic joints. Essential oil of lavender can be applied directly to the skin where it relieves most types of irritations and is particularly soothing for burns.

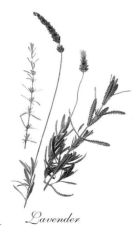

Lavender

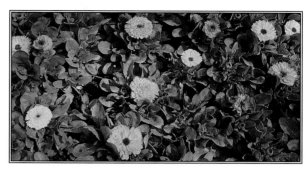

Marigold

MARIGOLD
Calendula officinalis

Part used: leaves, petals

History and mythology
This well-known flower opens and closes with the rising and setting of the sun. The marigold's old Saxon name was *ymbglidegold* meaning "that which moves round the sun". Its Latin name, *calendula*, refers to the belief that each plant blooms on the first day of the month in the Roman calendar. It was associated with clarity, energy, and harmony and with the constant and enduring rhythms of the planet Earth. By the twelfth century, those with poor eyesight or recurrent headaches were advised to gaze upon the bright marigold to improve their condition. The confused and bewildered, those the twentieth century would label stressed or suffering from burnout, were also advised to spend time looking at marigolds.

Harvesting and processing
Marigold petals are best gathered early in the morning when free from dew then spread thinly in an airy place to allow moisture to evaporate. Dry further in a dark place to preserve their color before storing in clean, dry containers.

Medicinal use
Marigold petals in a tincture or infusion will relieve anxiety, menstrual complaints, varicose veins, fevers, gastric, and digestive ailments. As an infusion used as a mouthwash, the herb treats ulcers, sore gums, or irritated eyes. As an ointment it eases sunburn, mild scalds, insect bites and stings, various skin inflammations, dry skin, and eczema. As a soothing oil, a compress, or as a decoction added to a footbath it will ease chilblains. Marigold oil or a decoction is added to bathwater to relieve stress generally. A marigold compress will also ease sprains, rheumatism, burns, and bruises. Marigold leaves applied to clean, shallow cuts, scratches, and grazes will rapidly staunch slight bleeding.

MARSHMALLOW
Althaea officinalis

Part used: leaves, roots

History and mythology
In ancient Greece, Hippocrates prescribed a decoction of marshmallow roots to treat bruises and loss of blood from severe wounds. The herb's botanical name comes from the Greek, *althos,* "to heal." Four centuries later, Dioscorides used marshmallow root poultices to relieve insect bites, toothache, vomiting, and as an antidote to poisons. In Arabia in the tenth century, physicians used anti-inflammatory poultices of mallow leaf. The confectionary is named after the flowers, which are rarely available commercially.

Harvesting and processing
Plants should be at least two years old before roots are harvested in autumn, when the top growth dies back and the mature tap root can be extracted from its bed. The lateral rootlets are removed before washing, peeling, and drying, either whole or sliced. To use the roots, chop finely, adding enough water to swell the root's spongy material (mucilage) to a gel.

Medicinal use
Marshmallow gel will help to heal cuts, scratches, scrapes, grazes and burns when applied directly to the site of injury. Taken internally as a decoction prepared from the crushed or chopped roots, marshmallow relieves an upset stomach, gastritis, peptic ulcers and the symptoms of upper and lower respiratory tract infections such as sore throats, coughs, colds, influenza, and bronchitis. An infusion of the leaves remedies bronchial and urinary disorders.

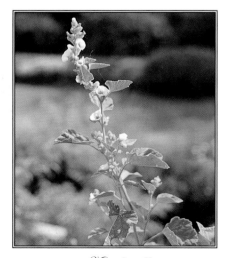

Marshmallow

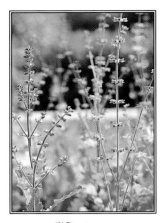

Meadowsweet

MEADOWSWEET
Filipendula ulmaria

Part used: leaves

History and mythology
In mediaeval Europe, meadowsweet's almond fragrance ensured its popularity as a strewing herb or air freshener. In the nineteenth century, German chemists became interested in meadowsweet when one discovered that its flower buds contained salicin, a powerful pain-reliever, fever-reducer, and anti-inflammatory. Others used an extract of meadowsweet to synthesize acetylsalicylic acid and called this new drug aspirin from the herb's old botanical name (*Spirea ulmaria*).

Harvesting and processing
Meadowsweet's leaves and large, drooping clusters of small, coiled flower tops are harvested when the plant is in bloom.

Medicinal use
As well as diuretic and sweat-inducing properties, meadowsweet is both an anti-inflammatory and an anti-acidic herb. As a natural source of salicylic acid, the base of aspirin, it offers all the benefits of that drug but because its other constituents — its oils, tannins, and minerals — soothe the digestion, meadowsweet does not irritate the gut as aspirin does and is used effectively to treat stomach and duodenal ulcers, heartburn, excess acidity, and indigestion. It is also prescribed, particularly as a compress, for rheumatism and arthritis. A mild tea of meadowsweet, drunk slowly three times daily, can relieve diarrhea in children but should never be given to children under two years nor to a child under 16 years of age if suffering fevers from colds, flu, or chicken pox. An infusion can also be used as a wash for eye irritations.

MINT

Mentha arvenis (field mint)
Mentha piperita (peppermint)
Mentha spicata (spearmint)
Mentha pulegium (pennyroyal)

Part used: leaves

History and mythology

Mints are recorded in the Ebers Papyrus, the world's oldest surviving medical text, and are frequently mentioned in the Bible. The Greeks and Romans crowned themselves with mint for banquets and put bunches of it on their tables to prevent drunkenness - in truth, Greek and Roman herbalists prescribed mint for just about everything, from hiccups to leprosy. The Romans introduced it to Britain and it was familiar to Chaucer and Shakespeare. Mint was valued as a strewing herb to perfume and repel insects in homes. The scientific name for pennyroyal, *mentha pulegium*, refers to the Latin *pulex* meaning flea. Ending a meal with a sprig of mint to help the digestion and sweeten the breath is a very ancient custom, culminating in the widespread popularity of today's chocolate-coated after-dinner mints. Field mint (*bo he*) is used mainly in Chinese medicine. In the West, herbalists prefer peppermint, spearmint, and pennyroyal.

Harvesting and processing

Growing stinging nettles near mint greatly increases the strength of peppermint's essential oil whereas chamomile nearby decreases the peppermint's but increases its own essential oil. Mint should be cut just before the fullness of flowering then bunched and hung until thoroughly dry, but no longer if the herb's potency is to be retained. To freeze, chop fresh leaves finely, scatter evenly in icecube trays and top with water; or wrap sprigs of fresh mint in sealed foil.

Medicinal use

Fresh or dried, peppermint leaf tea promotes sound sleep. Spearmint is usually preferred by children. Peppermint tea taken regularly throughout autumn and winter may help build resistance to colds. With its ability to promote sweating combined with its carminative, antispasmodic, and analgesic properties, mint will at least relieve cold symptoms as well as headaches, colic, flatulence, indigestion, and nausea. Sucking a mint candy or inhaling mint oil is a simple preventative or treatment for motion sickness. Mint inhalations may also relieve congestion. Applied topically, mint can ease inflammation and pain.

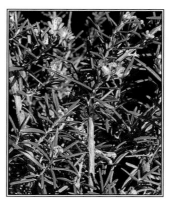

Rosemary

ROSEMARY

Rosmarinus offcinalis

Part used: leaves

History and mythology

Since ancient times rosemary has symbolized fidelity, love, and abiding friendship; it is still prescribed to strengthen memory and concentration as it stimulates blood flow to the brain. Rosemary has long been regarded as a preserver of youth; it is now known to be a powerful antioxidant. The herb is a very effective stimulant and was used in the attempts made to awaken the fairytale Sleeping Beauty. Bunches of rosemary were burned as protection against the plague; it has strong antiseptic, antibacterial, and antifungal properties, and it boosts the immune system.

Harvesting and processing

Use fresh at any time. For drying, branches are best cut before flowering, then hung in bunches in a shady, airy place. When dry, strip the leaves from the stalks. Sprays of fresh rosemary may be wrapped in foil, sealed, and frozen.

Medicinal use

There is in old saying that "Rosemary comforts the heart and quickens the spirit"; its warming and stimulating properties mean it is prescribed to increase vitality, soothe nervousness, counter fatigue, stimulate the kidneys, aid digestion and circulation, and improve appetite. A hot tea is good for colds and flu (it will promote sweating), and for rheumatism. Its expectorant, decongestant, and antispasmodic properties are an added boon to the treatment of bronchial and respiratory conditions. Rosemary is one of the best treatments for headache and migraine. A water or oil infusion as a rinse or a rub can help hair to shine, encourge growth, and counter dandruff. Rosemary is also reputed to strengthen sight.

RUE

Ruta graveolens

Part used: leaves

History and mythology

Rue originated in southern Europe and was introduced to Britain by the Romans. It is also known as the Herb of Grace, referring to a time when bunches of rue were used ceremonially to sprinkle holy water in the path of the priest as he approached the altar to say a High Mass. Rue was also said to defend its wearers against black magic and, conversely, to be an ingredient of witches' potions. Wild rue protected Ulysses from Circes' charm which transformed his men into swine.

Harvesting and processing

Just before flowering, cut rue plants near the base (they will shoot again), in the morning, after any dew has evaporated. Rue can be hung in loose bunches or spread to dry in the usual manner. Keep in mind that rue and basil are garden enemies.

Medicinal use

The taste of rue is extraordinarily bitter. Ancient and modern herbalists agree, however, on its potency in helping to remedy several maladies and that its use should be undertaken only by a qualified practitioner. Pregnant women are advised not to take rue. When prescribed accurately and taken exactly as directed, rue can relieve colic and indigestion, eliminate worms, and improve appetite. A rue ointment can help relieve the pain of sciatica, rheumatism, and gout. A liberal application of rue tea will repel flies and fleas from an area, including animals' coats, bedding, kennels, and baskets.

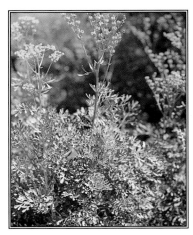

Rue

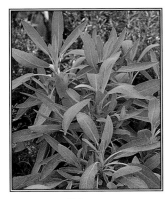

Sage

SAGE

Salvia officinalis

Part used: leaves

History and mythology

The Greek physician, Dioscorides, wrote of this herb as "Sage the Savior" and recommended it to ease headaches, nervous tension, and several internal complaints. The ancient Egyptians and the Chinese used sage as a brain tonic, and the English word "sage" remains synonymous with wisdom. The plant's scientific name is derived from the Latin *salvere*, a verb meaning "to be saved", and refers to the plant's reputation for preventative and curative powers. "He who would live for aye must eat sage in May" is an old English proverb and the recommendation of this herb for the elderly is fitting as it restores memory and energy, is helpful with many problems associated with menopause, restores color to grey hair, and is a powerful antioxidant.

Harvesting and processing

Harvest sage for drying just before the plant flowers. Sage can be bundled and hung or spread to dry in the usual way. Fresh sage leaves may also be chopped finely, put into icecube trays, covered with water and frozen. Note that sage and rosemary are mutually supportive in the garden.

Medicinal use

Sage benefits the liver and the digestive system. Sage infusions are highly antiseptic and astringent and can be applied as a compress to slow-healing wounds, or used as a gargle for throat and mouth problems, or as an inhalation for respiratory conditions. It also reduces perspiration. Sage provides a tonic to the nervous and female reproductive systems, and stimulates the immune system. In Chinese medicine, the root of *Salvia miltiorrhiza* (*dan shen*) is used.

SKULLCAP
Scutellaria laterifolia

Part used: leaves

History and mythology
American or Virginian skullcap is the one used by modern Western herbalists although Native Americans have long used it to treat rabies and promote menstruation. Eighteenth century European herbalists used skullcap to treat rabies, for insomnia and nervousness, recurring fevers, convulsions, and alcoholic delusions.

Harvesting and processing
Harvest the leaves of this herb late in the flowering period when the skull-shaped seed pods have appeared.

Medicinal use
This is one of the best tonics for the nervous system. An infusion of skullcap (honey or lemon will conceal its bitter taste) will combat nervous exhaustion, anxiety, and premenstrual tension, particularly symptomatic insomnia. Its antispasmodic properties make it useful for heart palpitations and epilepsy, and its anti-inflammatory action assists arthritis treatment. As a bitter herb it may help reduce fevers, enhance digestion, and stimulate the liver.

STINGING NETTLE
Urtica dioica

Part used: leaves

History and mythology
The Romans used to beat themselves with nettles to stay warm, and traditionally this activity has been used to relieve arthritis and rheumatism — the stinging hairs on the leaves contain formic acid and histamine which triggers an allergic response that was thought to be stimulating.

Harvesting and processing
Harvest while flowering. The leaves are particularly nourishing if gathered when young.

Medicinal use
As well as stimulating circulation, this highly nutritious plant contains iron, silica, and potassium, which makes it a good tonic for those convalescing or with anemia or arthritis (the Vitamin C content ensures the iron is properly absorbed). Nettles have an astringent action on the kidneys and bladder (helping cleanse the body of toxins), and on the blood (discouraging bleeding of all kinds). In juice, wash, or ointment form, nettles can alleviate skin problems, wounds, bites, and hemorrhoids, and is good for the hair.

Chinese herbalists use the root of Scutellaria baikalensis (huang quin) to clear heat from the respiratory and digestive systems, and as a sedative to calm convulsions.

ST JOHN'S WORT
Hypericum perforatum

Part used: flowers, leaves

History and mythology
The herb was thought to keep away evil and because an infusion of leaves was often used successfully as an equine remedy (although St John's wort or ragwort, like tansy, can be toxic to animals), it was named after St John, the patron saint of horses. Above all, St John's wort was believed to be a cure for the "ague", or malaria; a cure prescribed to the ancient Romans by Dioscorides and by Gerard and Culpeper to the people of sixteenth and seventeenth century England.

Harvesting and processing
St John's wort must be harvested when in flower. Flowerheads and leaves should be separated from the stems and allowed to dry before storing in clean, airtight containers. A hardy perennial, it is still found as a wild herb in field, meadow, and paddock.

Medicinal use
A tea of these leaves alleviates fever, depression, and insomnia, having a gently relaxing and restorative effect on the nervous system. Its mild analgesic effect may ease rheumatic, neuralgic, and sciatic pain. A poultice, an oil infusion, or an ointment made with the herb should relieve muscular strains, ease the discomfort of insect bites, and help heal skin damaged by cuts, grazes, bruises, or slight burns. St John' wort also has antibacterial, antiviral and expectorant actions. It is a diuretic, but has an astringent, antimicrobial effect on digestive problems like diarrhea.

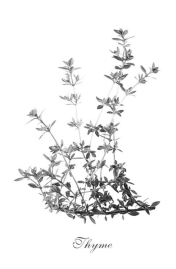

Thyme

THYME
Thymus vulgaris

Part used: leaves

History and mythology
The name of this herb may be a derivative of a Greek word meaning "to fumigate", or it may come from *thymus*, signifying courage. It is very much a summer herb, producing its strongest fragrance under the hottest sun, which draws out the aromatic oil. The Romans used thyme for digestion and as a remedy for "melancholy" — or hangovers. Thyme was commonly mentioned in early medical texts as an antiseptic, a decongestant, a respiratory treatment, and a digestive aid.

Harvesting and processing
Harvest the leafy branches just before flowering, early on a dry day. Thyme can be loosely bunched and hung or spread to dry in the usual manner. The taste and aroma of dried thyme is far stronger than fresh thyme. Washed and dried sprays of thyme can be sealed in foil and frozen.

Medicinal use
Thyme is a decongestant and expectorant with a relaxing and warming effect and has powerful antiseptic, antifungal, and astringent properties. It is valuable in treating coughs, colds, chest infections, sore throats, cramps, colic, diarrhea, poor digestion, and loss of appetite. Herbalists recommend thyme tea to relieve headaches, to cleanse and balance the bowel and bladder (it is an effective diuretic), and to tone the reproductive system. It is stimulating to the circulatory and immune systems and an excellent nerve tonic, helping to lift depression and relieve tension. Thyme is also said to improve the eyesight and clear the brain.

VALERIAN
Valeriana officinalis

Part used: roots

History and mythology
Dioscorides and Galen wrote of the powerful medicinal properties found in the root system of the plant they named Phu because of its strong smell. Valerian was widely used by Arab physicians in the tenth century, and by medieval monks in Europe. In some places, valerian still retains its country name of "all-heal". It has retained a reputation as a relaxing and soothing herb, a natural tranquillizer free of unpleasant side-effects.

Harvesting and processing
Stinging nettle grown as a companion plant increases the essential oil in valerian plants. To strengthen valerian roots, prune any flower buds. In autumn the green, leafy tops are cut away and the roots and rhizomes (rootstock) are collected. Brush off soil, dry and store in airtight containers.

Medicinal use
Valerian should be used under the guidance of a trained herbalist as a sedative and as an antispasmodic to ease irritating coughs, neuralgia, muscular cramps, and spasms. It assists in healing wounds and ulcers, and reducing blood pressure. The tea's strong taste improves with the addition of lemongrass. Respect the value of valerian tea: drink only in small quantities and over short periods of time.

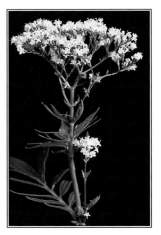

Valerian

Mugwort and wormwood are two closely related herbs, highly regarded in both Eastern and Western herbalism, particularly as bitter tonics to aid digestion.

MUGWORT and WORMWOOD
Artemisia vulgaris (mugwort)
Artemisia absinthium (wormwood)

Part used: flowers, leaves, roots

History and mythology
The herbs' scientific name comes from Artemis, the Greek name for Diana, Roman goddess of the hunt, who is said to have found this group of plants. Mugwort was also supposedly a witch's herb. In the Middle Ages, crystal-gazers claimed to employ the magnetic power of its north-turned leaves. Wormwood was hung in doorways to deflect evil spirits. It was also said to prevent intoxication, yet the leaves (which contain the potenially addictive thujone) are an ingredient in the highly intoxicating French liqueur, absinthe, and in bitter apertifs such as vermouth.

Harvesting and processing
It is preferable to gather these herbs in warm, dry weather, before noon, when the oil content of their leaves is at its richest, but they can be harvested successfully at any time of year. They can be bunched and hung or spread to dry in the usual way. Mugwort can be invasive and is more safely planted in pots. Wormwood can inhibit the growth of other plants; anise, fennel, sage, and caraway being especially vulnerable.

Medicinal use
Excessive use of these herbs can have adverse effects so they should be taken only with the advice of a professional herbalist.

Mugwort's dried, flowering shoots, leaves and roots are used in herbal medicine to ease menstrual difficulties, promote appetite and aid digestion. Wormwood's leaves, flowers, and roots also make an excellent general tonic, aid digestion, and expel worms.

YARROW
Achillea millefolium

Part used: flowers, leaves, stems

History and mythology
Yarrow has a number of descriptive folk names which indicate its ancient background and diverse uses. Achillea refers to the Greek hero Achilles who, legend says, treated his soldiers' battle wounds with this herb. Its pungent leaves were once prepared as snuff – accounting for another curious name it goes by: old man's pepper. Among yarrow's many other common names are staunch-weed, woundwort, nosebleed, and knight's mil-foil, all alluding to yarrow's reputation for staunching blood. It is still used in modern remedies for this purpose.

Harvesting and processing
Harvest the entire plant, other than the roots, in late summer when in full bloom, on a sunny day after any dew has evaporated but before the full heat of the day. Bunch and hang or spread to dry in usual way. When dry, separate flowers and set aside. Strip leaves from stalks, crumble and set aside. Finely chop stems. Then recombine all parts. Some herbal remedies call for fresh leaves.

Medicinal use
Yarrow tea, made from the whole plant, has a powerful tonic effect on the system helping to allay fevers, purify the blood, lift depression, and treat kidney disorders. It promotes sweating and is recommended for treating colds and flu. When used as a wash, it is said to prevent baldness. The fresh leaves are sometimes made into an ointment, a poultice, or an infusion to apply to wounds. The flowers are transformed by steam into an anti-allergin. Respiratory and digestive problems also respond to yarrow which can also be used, under supervision, for menstrual difficulties and for staunching blood. Yarrow tea is best saved for obvious, remedial use only because frequent or unwarranted use can produce unpleasant side effects.

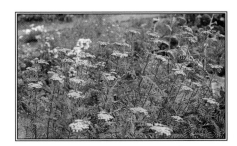

Yarrow

Using herbs

*One of the advantages of the more simple
herbal treatments, particularly when used for less complex
health conditions, is that you can safely prepare
many of them at home.*

There are herbal treatments that should be prescribed by a herbalist, and others that can be self-prescribed. The most common forms are:
• Teas made by steeping flowers, berries, leaves, stems and other, usually soft, plant material in boiling water.
• Infusions are similar to teas but the herbs are steeped longer, in hot or cold oil or hot water, so that they are stronger than teas.
• Decoctions made by bringing herbs and water to the boil and simmering slowly to extract the natural herbal essences, and more often from the harder material such as the roots and bark of the plant.
• Tinctures made by extracting herbal essences by steeping the herb in alcohol or vinegar (wine or apple cider vinegar but not white vinegar).
• Compresses applied by repeated topical application of tea, decoction, or diluted tincture using soft, preferably cotton cloth (see page 47).
• Poultices of crushed, ground, heated, soaked, or boiled herbs which are applied directly to the skin or on a dressing (see page 49).
• Inhalations of steam rising from a mixture of boiling water poured over a herb or herbs (see page 48).
• Herbal tablets or capsules. Measured, powdered herbs can be divided and packed into standard, commercially available gelatin capsules to allow for correct dosage prescription and easy portability and consumption.

• Concentrated liquid medication (perhaps a tincture or decoction) absorbed by placing drops under the tongue.
• Ointments, oils and lotions in which herbs are steeped directly or into which herbal infusions, decoctions or tinctures are added.

Whatever your chosen form of self-treatment, if your condition does not start to improve gradually after a few weeks, consult a herbalist.

Infusions and teas

There is no easier way to introduce health-promoting herbs into your daily life than preparing your own herbal infusions (much more than just a caffeine-free alternative to tea or coffee). The recipes in this book provide safe doses for their regular consumption.

Herbal infusions, also known as tisanes, are teas made by infusing or steeping leaves, flowers, bark, seeds, berries, or roots in water. They may be enjoyed at any time but moderation is advisable and a balanced intake of different herb teas rather than an emphasis on one or another is the healthiest approach to their use.

Information about the preventative and healing focus of different teas is outlined in Herbal Infusions on page 42.

There are many teas available commercially or you may choose to make your own infusions using the instructions here as a basis.

The addition of extra water to dilute the tea, honey or fruit to sweeten, or yeast extract to give extra flavor are acceptable additives.

A cupful is generally taken three to six times daily, depending on the severity of the condition.

Usually, teas are drunk hot, except when treating the urinary system when they should be consumed lukewarm or cool.

Some herbs with a high mucilage content (a gel-like substance) should be prepared using cold water.

Infusions should be made fresh daily but can be kept in the refrigerator for up to two days.

One more tip: Keep a separate teapot for your herbal teas, whether homemade or commercially prepared.

When a a weak tea or infusion is desired, the following quantities are suitable: half to one teaspoon dried or one and a half to three teaspoons fresh herb to one cup (8 fl oz/ 250 ml) of boiling water.

When a strong tea or infusion is wanted, an effective ratio is 1 oz (30 g) dried or 3 oz (90 g) fresh to 16 fl oz (500 ml) of boiling water.

Leaf teas

Pour 1 cup of water boiled in a non-aluminum container over 1 teaspoon of dried or 3 teaspoons of fresh herbs in a small teapot or jug. Allow the leaves to infuse for about 3 minutes before pouring and straining into a cup.

Flower teas or infusions

Use 1 teaspoon of fresh flowerheads or petals or 3 teaspoons of dried, per cup of water. Bring water to the boil in a non-aluminum saucepan, add the flowerheads or petals, cover, simmer for 1 minute and stand for 3 minutes before pouring and straining the infusion.

Root teas

Root teas (valerian is one) are made in the same way as leaf teas but with roots which have been thoroughly washed, sliced, and dehydrated before being placed in a kitchen blender to be ground to either a granular or powdery consistency, depending on the plant.

Seed teas

When making teas from the seeds of plants, for instance aniseed tea, the seeds should be crushed first to release their medicinal oils and the tea should stand a few minutes more than most teas before being poured through a strainer.

Make a tonic wine by covering 1 lb (500 g) of herb with 64 fl oz (2 L) of red wine. Seal and leave for two weeks. Take in sherry glass doses. This works particularly well for roots like ginger or ginseng.

Decoctions

These are basically the same as infusions but are made from the harder parts of a plant, such as the bark, roots, rhizomes, or nuts, and so need extra time and heat to brew.

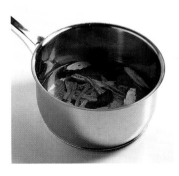 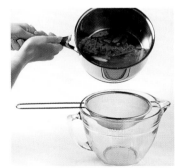

1. Place the chopped or sliced herb in a pan with water (in the same proportion as for infusions but with a little extra water to allow for evaporation).

2. Bring water to boil, cover, and simmer for 10 minutes. Strain liquid before using.

Hot oil infusion

A hot infusion can be made from soft plant material such as leaves, flowers, and berries and is used in massage oils or added to ointments and lotions. Store in clean, airtight, dark glass bottles.

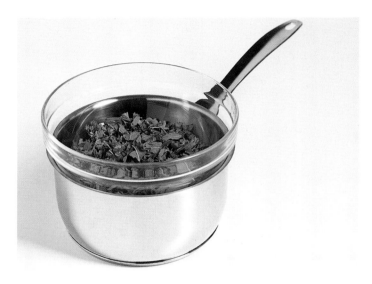

1. Place 8 oz (250 g) dried or 24 oz (750 g) fresh herb and 16 fl oz (500 ml) vegetable oil in a glass bowl over a saucepan or in a non-aluminum double saucepan containing simmering water and heat on low for 3 hours.

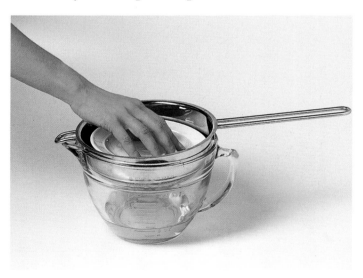

2. Strain the mixture through a fine sieve or through muslin or cheesecloth, squeezing out as much liquid as possible (you can push down with a plate if using a sieve, or wring out the fabric).

Cold oil infusion

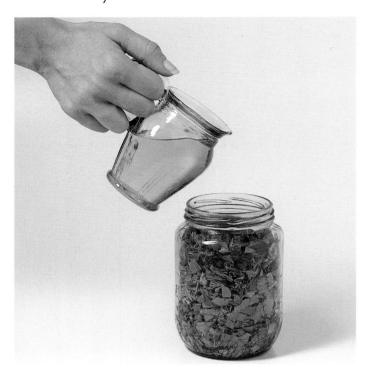

1. Pack herbs into a large jar and cover completely with oil. Seal and leave in a sunny place for two to three weeks.

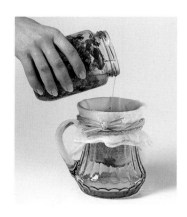

2. Strain the mixture through muslin or cheesecloth. Coffee filter paper can also be used but straining will be slower.

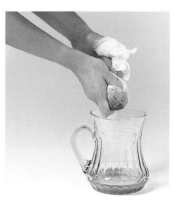

3. Squeeze out as much liquid as possible. Use this strained oil to pour into another large jar packed with more herb. Let stand as before and strain again. Repeat the soaking and straining process for a third time. Transfer product of final infusion to clean, airtight, dark glass bottles. Store in a cool, dark place.

Never hesitate to eat culinary herb flowers, fresh or dried, as well as the leaves. The two blend beautifully together.

Tinctures

Tinctures are herbal concentrates that involve steeping fresh or dried herbs in alcohol and water. This extracts the plant's active ingredients and the alcohol acts as a preservative so that tinctures can be kept for up to two years. Vodka is recommended due to its relative purity, although brandy, rum, or gin can also be used.

The usual dose is one teaspoon of tincture diluted in water and consumed with or after food, three times daily. Children should be given half this dose, and toddlers only a quarter. Tinctures can also be used as gargles, mouthwashs, and as a herbal lotion or wash.

It is important to use the right quantity of alcohol. This may look complicated at first but it isn't — just follow the equation below.

First make up a mixture that is 25 per cent (one-quarter) consumable alcohol to 75 per cent (three-quarters) water. To do so, you must know the alcoholic content of the liquor you are using; this is usually noted on the bottle's label, perhaps with the word "proof". Vodka, for instance, is usually labelled approximately 40 per cent alcohol and 60 per cent water. This will obviously need to be diluted further to make up the correct proportion. To do this, it is usually easiest to make up 32 fl oz (1 L), and use one of the equations below as a formula (adjusting for whatever alcohol you are using):

Imperial

8 fl oz (ie 25 per cent of 1 litre) x 100 ÷ 40
(ie alcohol percentage of vodka) = 20 fl oz
To make 32 fl oz of tincture base, add 12 fl oz vodka
and 20 fl oz water.

Metric

250 ml (ie 25 per cent of 1 litre) x 100 ÷ 40
(ie alcohol percentage of vodka) = 625 ml
To make 1 litre of tincture base, add 375 ml vodka
and 625 ml water.

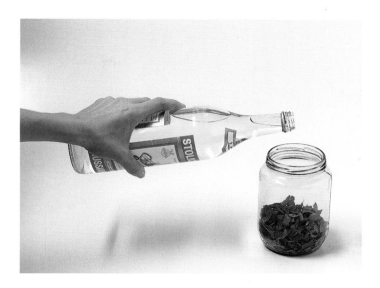

1. Place 8 oz (250 g) dried herb or 16 oz (500 g) fresh herbs in a large jar and cover with the alcohol/water mixture. Seal the jar and store in a cool place for 2 to 6 weeks, shaking occasionally to encourage the alcohol to absorb the herb's medicinal constituents. If the liquid level subsides, replace with more alcohol or vinegar.

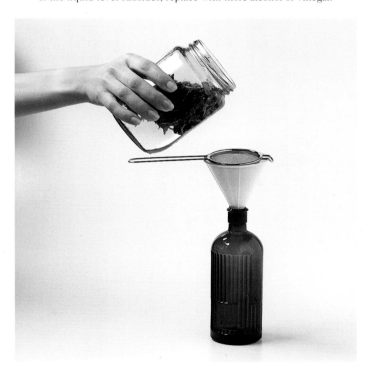

2. Strain the mixture through a sieve or through muslin or cheesecloth. Store in clean, airtight, dark glass bottles in a cool, dark place.

Herbal Infusions

Making your own herbal infusions or teas is easy —
just look to page 38 for details. Teas should be made fresh daily.

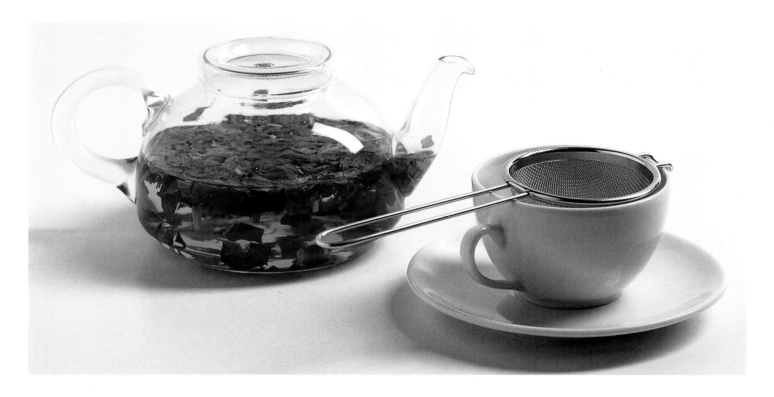

Combination herbal brews

Two teas may be mixed, especially if the tastes are complementary and their beneficial effects differ. No milk is added to herb teas (the exception being slippery elm bark tea). Honey, a squeeze of lemon, orangeflower water, or rosewater (available from health food stores and delicatessens) may be added to taste. In summer, icecubes, stalks of fresh leafy herbs, and a little mineral water or fresh fruit juice, transform chilled herbal teas into refreshing, cool, and healthy drinks.

Angelica tea

A tea made from angelica's fresh or dried leaves is excellent for colds and influenza or soothing the nerves. The pleasant-tasting leaves are ideal mixers with less palatable herbs. The bruised root produces a tea which relieves flatulence. The addition of angelica leaf tea to a hot bath will add fragrance and increase relaxation.

Aniseed tea

One of the seed teas, aniseed tea is helpful in allaying colds and relieving indigestion and flatulence. Small amounts of powdered aniseed added to their food will help young children's digestion. Added to warm milk and honey, it will help soothe a fretful child. Aniseed tea freshens the palate, sweetens the breath, and brightens the eyes. It is also used as a lotion to lighten the skin.

Basil leaf tea

A tea of basil leaves (which combine well with borage leaves) is good for the lungs and diseases of the kidneys and bladder. Basil leaves infused in wine and patted onto the face helps to close enlarged pores.

Bay leaf tea

A tea of bay leaves is excellent for the digestion and is somewhat astringent as well (see details on facial steaming on page 52).

Bergamot leaf tea

This tea can be used as a remedy for sore throats and chest complaints. Add to a hot bath for a revitalizing, pleasantly perfumed soak.

Borage leaf tea

A tea of borage is used as a heart tonic, as a stimulant for the adrenal glands, and as a systemic purifier. Mixed with basil it assists the kidneys and bladder, heart and glands, as well as generally strengthening the system.

Caraway seed tea

This seed combines well with borage leaf and is beneficial to the digestive and elimination systems, relieving flatulence and clearing the complexion.

Chamomile flower tea

This is one of the best-known herb teas, long used as a soothing beverage and especially effective when taken before sleep. German chamomile flowers are considered more potent than other varieties. A cup of chamomile tea is recommended for menstrual pain and nervous tension. A very weak chamomile tea with honey calms young children who are teething or simply overtired.

Chervil leaf tea

Chervil has always been valued as a blood purifier. The tea also helps the kidneys, brightens dull eyes, and clears the complexion. Chervil tea compresses will help reduce swellings and bruises.

Chicory root tea or coffee

This tea is excellent when recovering from a bilious attack or from hepatitis, and is generally good for the liver and gall bladder. It also has laxative and diuretic properties. However, it is not recommended for people who are anemic.

Chive leaf tea

A tea made from chopped fresh chive leaves will stimulate the appetite, prove a tonic for the kidneys, lower blood pressure and, because chives are a source of calcium, help to strengthen nails and teeth.

Comfrey leaf tea

Comfrey tea is an old country remedy for healing internal injuries and broken bones. It contains a large amount of calcium and vitamin B12 so promotes the formation of strong teeth and bones. It also aids the circulation, cleanses the bloodstream and is said to benefit those suffering from ulcers caused by varicose veins.

Poultices soaked in strong comfrey tea can be applied to injured muscles and areas of bone weakness.

Coriander seed tea

Tea made from coriander seeds is excellent for the digestion, relieving gripe pain and flatulence. It is another herb tea used traditionally to purify the blood and thus clear the complexion.

Cress leaf tea

All cresses, especially watercress, are rich in vitamins and minerals, containing sulphur, iron, iodine, and phosphorus. Cress tea, a natural blood purifier, is excellent for clearing the complexion and brightening the eyes. Beside making one more robust, cress tea is said to help prevent hair loss. Parsley combines well with cress in tea.

Dandelion coffee

This beverage is made from the roots of wild dandelions and is commonly packaged and sold in powdered or granulated form. Check that no unhealthy additives have been used to counter the dandelion's natural, slightly bitter taste. By stimulating the liver and urinary tract, dandelion tea helps to prevent rheumatism and similar complaints.

Dill seed tea

Very weak, dill seed tea, made with boiling water but given lukewarm, may help a baby's colic. In adults, stronger dill tea helps the digestion and dispels flatulence. It is also reputed to strengthen the fingernails.

Elderflower tea

A tea made from the fresh or dried blooms of the elder tree is an old remedy for influenza and for purifying the blood.

*Many herb teas
also make excellent
skin lotions.
The infusion is first
cooled and then lightly
patted onto the face and
neck with moistened
cotton or tissue.*

Fennel seed tea

As well as relieving indigestion and helping to rid the body of uncomfortable gases, cooled fennel seed tea is excellent for bathing sore eyes.

Lemon balm tea

This tea helps to reduce high temperatures as it induces perspiration. It also lessens the effects of exhaustion in hot weather, assists the appetite and the digestion, helps to settle an upset stomach, eases gripe, and is an anti-depressant. Double-strength lemon balm tea in a hot bath cleanses and perfumes the skin.

Lemongrass leaf tea

This is one of the most palatable of all herb teas. Being rich in vitamin A, it encourages clear, smooth textured skin.

Lime flower tea or linden tea

The fresh or dried flowers from the large lime tree, *Tilia europaea*, make a fragrant tea which may be taken regularly as a general tonic, and which is also known to calm the nerves and soothe the mucous linings disturbed by upper respiratory tract infections such as head colds.

Lovage tea

The leaves of lovage make an excellent digestive tea. The cooled tea also makes a soothing lotion for sore eyes. The root of the lovage plant is sometimes used to make a tea to assist jaundice and bladder problems. A tea made from the seeds is recommended as a gargle for mouth and throat infections.

Marjoram and oregano tea

A brew of marjoram and oregano leaves at the onset of a fever helps induce beneficial perspiration. It also relieves colds, cramps, digestive troubles, nervous headaches, and stomach pains. Marjoram or oregano leaves plus flowers, produce a tea which has both a tonic and a soothing effect.

Mint leaf tea

Peppermint tea is the best known of mint teas which are particularly refreshing served cold. It is a carminative tea, meaning it disperses congestion in the body to relieve indigestion, bronchitis, headaches, coughs, and colds. Tea made from spearmint leaves is also good for the digestion, cleansing the intestines, helping to dispel stomach gases, and eliminating bad breath.

Nettle leaf tea

A tea made from the dried leaves of the common nettle contains vitamin D, iron, calcium, and other important trace elements and is used as a blood tonic. It is taken in cases of arterial degeneration, rheumatism, gout, and shortness of breath. The leaves, fresh or dried, also make a delicious and nutritious soup.

Slippery elm bark tea

This highly nutritious tea comes from the bark of a small tree, *Ulmus fulva*, native to the United States and Canada. The inner bark of the trunk and larger branches is dried and powdered.

Into a cup, place a teaspoon of slippery elm powder, a pinch of cinnamon, and enough cold water to mix to a paste. Stir briskly while adding very hot but not boiling water or milk plus a teaspoon of clear honey. When brewed, slippery elm powder produces a very glutinous beverage. Should the mixture be lumpy, press it through a fine sieve.

Slippery elm tea's lack of visual appeal is outweighed by its power to strengthen and heal generally and particularly to soothe the intestines. It can make some people sleepy, so is best imbibed before bedtime or when one is free to doze.

*If using fresh herbs
for tea,
use twice the quantity
than for dried,
and infuse for several
minutes longer.*

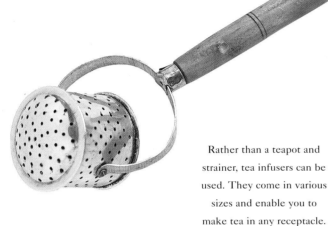

Rather than a teapot and
strainer, tea infusers can be
used. They come in various
sizes and enable you to
make tea in any receptacle.

Parsley leaf tea

Parsley is a very nutritious herb, containing vitamins A, B, and C, as well as organic iron, potassium, silicon, magnesium, and other trace elements. It should, however, be avoided by pregnant women. This tea stimulates the appetite, is a tonic and a cleanser, assisting the bladder, kidneys, and liver, and is excellent for people suffering from anemia. It is also helpful, with other treatment, in overcoming chronic cystitis. Parsley and watercress tea blend well.

Raspberry leaf tea

Dried raspberry leaf tea traditionally was given to pregnant women because it was reputed to ease childbirth and the expulsion of the afterbirth, promote lactation, and hasten convalescence. A soothing tea, it tones the mucous membranes, allays nausea, and promotes a healthy bowel.

Rosehip tea

The hip is actually the fruit of the rose. Many people swear that rosehip tea — an excellent source of vitamins A, C, E, and B — prevents colds. It strengthens the lungs to fight infection and is particularly useful for those with chronic chest problems. Rosehips have an uplifting, restorative effect on the nervous system and can assist with insomnia, fatigue, and irritability. Try adding a little honey and pinch of spice. In summer, iced rosehip tea may be pepped up with sprigs of mint or peppermint, honey or lemon. Fragrant hibiscus flowers blend well with rosehips in tea.

Rosemary leaf tea

This tea is recommended for strengthening the memory and relieving headaches, as a nerve tonic, and to aid the kidneys and the digestive system generally.

Sage leaf tea

The ancient Egyptians and Chinese were aware of the properties of this tea which promotes longevity, strengthens memory, restores acuteness to the senses and benefits the liver, brain, and nerves. It is excellent when blended with lemon balm. The cooled tea soothes as a mouth rinse for inflamed gums and as a gargle for sore throats.

Savory leaf tea

Savory is an intestinal antiseptic and is also said to be an aphrodisiac. Both winter and summer savory make pleasant teas used to treat colic, flatulence, giddiness, and respiratory troubles.

Tarragon leaf tea

Herbalists recommend tarragon tea to ease indigestion and flatulence. By acting as a diuretic, it helps to rid the body of excess fluids.

Thyme leaf tea

Take this tea as an aid to digestion and to tone up the nervous system and respiratory organs. It is also an intestinal antiseptic.

Valerian root tea

This tea, while not habit-forming, has remarkable sedative properties, soothing and calming the nerves. It also relieves migraine and heart palpitations. It should be taken just before bedtime. Some herbal therapists advise people suffering from liver complaints against valerian tea as it can cause nausea. If you find its scent unpleasant, it may be mixed with a more pleasant herb such as lemongrass, or honey or fruit juice can be added.

Healing with Herbs

Herbalists prescribe simple or compound herbal treatments to help heal the body by assisting it to remove toxic or waste products, to ease distressing symptoms, to trigger the body's own healing mechanisms, and to build healthy organs, blood, and tissue.

If you have a longstanding or chronic health problem such as asthma, arthritis, eczema or acne, herbal treatment is best thought of in terms of months rather than weeks and ideally should be monitored by a trained herbalist. When wellbeing has been achieved and remains constant for approximately two to three months, your herbalist might review and adjust your medication to a maintenance dosage. In the worst cases, where the body has sustained permanent damage over many years, the best a herbalist can achieve might be relief rather than remedy.

We all know that our bodies are highly individual organisms; that some seem to thrive on a few hours sleep where others need a regular eight hours; that some can tolerate alcohol or coffee where others can't; that some shrug off a cold but suffer crippling migraine headaches. Herbalism is able to respond to our different needs in terms of dosages or forms of medication we find more acceptable. Some of us might find strong-tasting drops under the tongue appealing while those who would find them appalling would delight in preparing and slowly sipping a curative herbal tea.

For information about making your own herbal remedies, see Using Herbs on page 38. Tinctures with the correct balance of herbs can be purchased commercially.

Herbal remedies can and do offer immediate relief or remedy to conditions that usually have a short duration; ailments such as coughs, colds, and sore throats, for example. If self-treating these minor conditions, it's wise to continue your herbal remedies for a minimum of three days after the last sign of any symptom.

With conditions such as bronchitis or sinusitis where the worst can be over in a few days or where they continue for longer than we feel appropriate or quickly recur, herbal treatments tend to produce subtle but cumulative change for the better in the course of consistent treatment over some weeks.

Peppermint travel pillow

To ease apprehension and motion sickness fill a small sachet with:

2 oz (50 g) peppermint

1/2 oz (15 g) mint-scented pelargonium

2 oz (50 g) lemon verbena

2 oz (50 g) lavender

1 tablespoon crushed lemon zest

1 teaspoon crushed nutmeg chips

5 to 6 drops peppermint oil

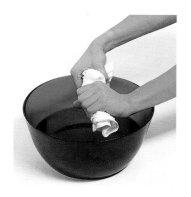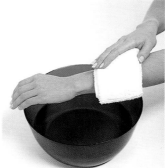

Compress

A compress consists of a soft cloth
moistened with herbal solution and applied
to the site of discomfort.
An infusion, decoction, or diluted tincture
may be gently pre-heated until
comfortable to touch, although cool liquid
is used for some conditions like headaches.
Soak a piece of absorbent cotton or surgical
gauze in the liquid, squeezing out any
excess before applying to the affected area.

Acne
Dandelion can reduce acne because it helps the liver
remove toxins from the body. Try drinking two cups of
dandelion tea per day. Other helpful, blood-purifying herbs
are: burdock, clivers, echinacea, marigold, red clover, and
yellow dock.

Anxiety
Valerian, skullcap, and hops will calm anxiety. Slowly sip
15 drops each of oats and passionflower tinctures in 1 cup
of water as often as required.

Arthritis
Guaiacum is a specifically anti-arthritic herb.
Meadowsweet's alkaline action assists arthritis sufferers by
normalizing gut acidity, dandelion and greater celandine by
their beneficial action on the liver, black cohosh and wild
yam by relieving pain, celery by countering the fluid
retention accompanying swelling. Herbal ointment
containing rue promotes pain relief when rubbed for about
30 minutes at least once a day into those parts of the body
affected by arthritis.

Asthma
Herbs specifically for asthma include lobelia and grindelia.
Comfrey and coltsfoot are also prime herbs for this
condition. Others which help to reduce lung infections
include echinacea, elecampane and wild cherry bark.

Back pain
Massage for 30 minutes daily with herbal ointment
containing rue to relieve pain and spasm in strained back
muscles.

Bladder disorders
Buchu tea is an antiseptic herbal remedy which cleanses
the urinary system and helps to relieve most bladder
dysfunctions, including cystitis and incontinence.
Try drinking 2 cups of buchu tea per day. The herbs
bearberry (commonly known as uva ursi), corn silk, and
slippery elm powder also assist with cystitis.

Body odor
A mixture of 10 to 15 drops of gentian tincture in 1 cup of
water taken 3 times daily before meals counters poor food
absorption, a possible cause of unpleasant body odor.

Bronchitis
Coltsfoot is generally the herbalist's herb of choice for
bronchitis. Other useful herbs include hyssop, echinacea,
golden seal, wild cherry bark, and elecampane.

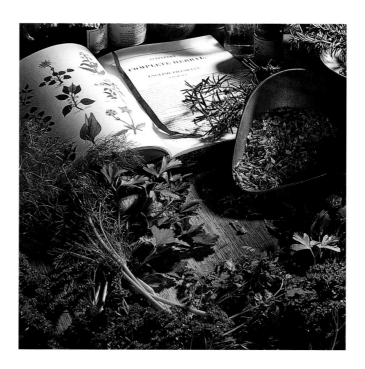

Steam inhalations can help relieve cold symptoms.

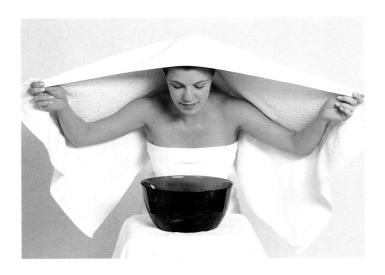

Burns
The pain of burns, including sunburn, can be significantly relieved by aloe vera, a great analgesic and healer. Apply aloe vera leaf gel three times daily for about 30 minutes. Once burn wounds have closed, comfrey ointment can help reduce scarring.

Chapped skin
Marigold and comfrey ointment used twice daily reduces skin dryness. The essential fatty acids of evening primrose oil are also good for the skin.

Chilblains
Prickly ash and ginger in the autumn protect against winter chilblains and drinking 1 cup of ginger tea night and morning may help reduce them. Chili in food is also said to prevent chilblains.

Colds and flu
Herbalists counter colds with warmth. Herbs to heat the body are: peppermint, chili, yarrow, and elder in the early stages and ginger and prickly ash if a cold lingers. Drink peppermint tea 3 times daily. Other beneficial herbs are echinacea and golden seal for infection, hyssop and coltsfoot for cough, eyebright and elder for sinus, golden rod to reduce mucus, and boneset for aches and pains. Tablets are available that contain a combination of these herbs.

Cold sores
If applied early and often, an ointment of the herb bittersweet will help prevent the growth of a cold sore. If the sore becomes wet and active apply solanum nigrum oil instead.

Colitis
Slippery elm bark is used to relieve all infections of the bowel. Add one teaspoon of slippery elm bark powder to a few spoonfuls of hot water, mix to a paste, add hot water or milk and drink immediately. Do so two to three times a day. Marshmallow and the astringent herbs cranesbill, agrimony, and wild yam may be prescribed preventively.

Constipation
Slippery elm bark is often prescribed for constipation as are aloe, bearberry, cascara sagrada, rhubarb root, senna pods, and yellow dock.

Corns
Before going to bed, crush a comfrey leaf in your hands until it becomes moist, then place over the corn and cover it with an old sock. Repeat over a few nights and the corn will disappear very quickly. A poultice mash of equal parts of roasted onion and soft soap is also recommended.

Cuts and scratches
Commercially available herbal creams contain marigold, comfrey, and St John's wort to heal cuts and scratches. Apply to clean wounds and cover. If a wound is dirty, apply an antiseptic cream containing St John's wort.

Dandruff
Rub chickweed lotion into the scalp before bedtime and next morning wash the hair with chickweed shampoo.

Depression
Herbs generally prescribed to treat depression include balm, St John's wort, valerian, oats, skullcap, and passionflower. Twice daily, drink a cup of tea made with one or more of these herbs.

Diarrhea
Slippery elm is the best herb for diarrhea while barley water prevents dehydration. For a temporary bout of diarrhea take one teaspoon of slippery elm powder every two hours until symptoms subside. Mix it with honey and banana to make it palatable unless the fruit aggravates the symptoms.

Eczema

Chickweed soothes eczema most effectively. For a dry, scaly but non-itchy eczema rash, apply a greasy form of chickweed ointment twice daily. For a red, itchy, eczema rash, apply sorbolene-based chickweed cream. For a violently hot itchy eczema rash, apply chickweed tincture with equal parts of water. Chronic eczema can be also treated internally with burdock and yellow dock.

Fluid retention

Herbs which are often prescribed for fluid retention include dandelion leaf, celery, buchu, and bearberry. These can be taken in teas or as tincture depending on the diagnosed cause and extent of the condition.

Gall bladder discomfort

The best home remedy for gall bladder distress is the addition of fresh lemon or lemon juice and olive oil to meals, especially to salads.

Gingivitis

To relieve the discomfort of sore gums, gargle twice daily with a mixture of equal parts of thyme, sage, and myrrh tinctures with glycerine (to coat exposed surfaces) in a glass of water.

Hemorrhoids

Witchhazel, marigold, comfrey, horse-chestnut, cranesbill, and oak bark can be taken internally, dabbed on externally, or used in a cream to ease the symptoms of hemorrhoids.

Hayfever

Garlic and horseradish tablets may reduce hayfever by strengthening the immune system. Other helpful herbs are echinacea, elder, eyebright, and golden seal.

Headaches

Depending on the cause of the headache, chamomile, feverfew, hops, wood betony, rosemary, fringetree, vervain, meadowsweet, and jamaican dogwood may bring relief. If a headache is stress-related, valerian, skullcap, and oats may be prescribed. Tea made from chamomile, meadowseet, or both should relieve a mild headache.

High blood pressure

Adding garlic, especially raw garlic, to the diet may help reduce blood pressure. Herbalists often prescribe hawthorn berries, lime blossom, oats, nettle, motherwort, and damiana for this condition and valerian, skullcap, and passionflower are also used to induce relaxation.

Poultice

Similar to a compress in that herbs are applied directly but as a healing paste to distressed parts of the body such as aching muscles, bruises, and arthritic joints.

Poultices also relieve troublesome skin infections by encouraging discharge from pimples, boils, and abscesses.

Poultices should never be used where skin is broken because any harmful bacteria present will thrive in response to the moist, warm poultice.

If fresh herbs are used, the quantity depends on the body area to be covered. For beginners, remember that a large bunch of herbs shrinks before your eyes once chopped finely.

If fresh herbs aren't available, first use dried herbs to prepare a decoction (see page 39). Powders can be mixed with water to form a paste.

Chop fresh herbs and place in a non-aluminum saucepan. Barely cover with water, bring to the boil and simmer for a few minutes before cooling until comfortable to the touch.

Then thoroughly strain the liquid and reserve the herbs. If the herbs are inclined to separate, bind them by adding a little slippery elm powder.

To prevent the poultice sticking to the skin, first spread or brush a thin layer of oil onto the affected area. Now spread a layer of the herbal paste and cover with clean gauze, a bandage or a strip of cotton or linen. Leave the poultice in place while resting the body for at least 30 minutes.

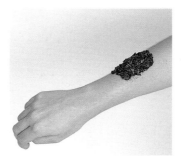
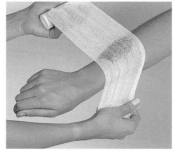

Hives

If you experience regular bouts of hives, nettle ointment applied to them twice daily will reduce inflammation and irritation.

Indigestion

Herbs prescribed for this condition include meadowsweet, fennel, dill, ginger, agrimony, chamomile, cinnamon, valerian, oats, skullcap, and gentian. A teaspoon measure of meadowsweet tincture in a little milk after each meal should relieve indigestion and may be repeated 30 minutes later if necessary.

Insomnia

To bring about relaxed, uninterrupted sleep, before going to bed take 10 drops each of jamaican dogwood, valerian, and passionflower tinctures in half a cup of water. If disturbed during the night, the same dosage may be repeated. Hyssop with chamomile and lavender flowers, valerian root, and peppermint leaves also makes a sedative bedtime tea. Skullcap and hops are also known to be sedative herbs.

Laryngitis

A tender larynx will respond well to a gargle made from an infusion of sage, thyme, and myrrh, plus a teaspoon of glycerine to coat the throat lining. Three times daily.

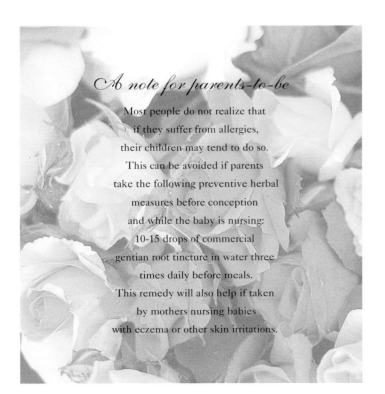

A note for parents-to-be

Most people do not realize that
if they suffer from allergies,
their children may tend to do so.
This can be avoided if parents
take the following preventive herbal
measures before conception
and while the baby is nursing:
10-15 drops of commercial
gentian root tincture in water three
times daily before meals.
This remedy will also help if taken
by mothers nursing babies
with eczema or other skin irritations.

Menopause

Herbs to relieve the symptoms of menopause include black cohosh, chaste tree, and false unicorn root to balance and stabilize hormone levels. St John's wort remedies the anxiety which is often symptomatic of the menopause. Motherwort and sage relieve hot flushes. Regular consumption of sage tea is recommended throughout this natural life process.

Migraines

Feverfew tea, dandelion, fringetree, vervain, ginger, valerian, cramp bark, wood betony, and jamaican dogwood have all been employed successfully to treat migraine headache.

Muscle cramps

A daily cup of tea made from wild yam, cramp bark, prickly ash, and black cohosh can reduce cramp by increasing circulation and relaxing tense muscles. If cramps are worse at night, drink the tea just before bedtime. This herbal combination is also available in tablet form.

Nausea

Chamomile, cinnamon, fennel, marshmallow, dill, meadowsweet, and peppermint are used to treat nausea. Black horehound is especially beneficial if used fresh from the garden, and is particularly effective for morning sickness in the form of tea made from a 2 inch (5 cm) stem of the herb steeped in a cup of hot water. If vomiting has occurred, peppermint will settle the stomach. If no vomiting has occurred, the body will probably tolerate and benefit from ginger tablets or ginger tea.

Nosebleeds

Apply a cold compress of yarrow to the nose and allow it to rest until well after bleeding has stopped.

Pain

Pain-relieving herbs include black cohosh, hops, and cramp bark. Other calming herbs are valerian, skullcap, and oats. Muscular pain responds to a thoroughly penetrating, 30-minute rub with rue ointment.

Period pain

To reduce abdominal pain and tension, mix 24 drops of chaste tree tincture with 6 drops of marigold tincture in a glass of water and drink three times daily for five days preceding the onset of menstruation.

Sciatica

Analgesic herbs which help to relieve sciatica include
St John's wort, black cohosh, jamaican dogwood, marigold,
and yarrow. Apply rue ointment to the skin three times
daily for deep pain, massaging for 30 minutes to allow it
to penetrate.

Shingles

Mix 5 drops of St John's wort tincture and 5 drops of
vervain tincture in a glass of water and drink hourly.
To relieve acute distress, equal parts of St John's wort
tincture, plantain tincture, and water may be applied
directly to the skin as often as required. Later, St John's
wort ointment may be applied to the rash.

Sinusitis

Commercially available teas contain echinacea, horseradish,
and garlic to combat the infection; marshmallow and
comfrey to soothe irritation and soreness; the astringents
golden seal and eyebright; chamomile, peppermint, hyssop,
ginger, and cinnamon to loosen mucus. Three cups daily
are usually recommended. Echinacea tablets and ones
containing a combination of garlic and horseradish will also
strengthen the immune system against future infection.

Stomach ache

If the stomach ache is due to indigestion, gentian in
tincture form is the herb to take. If this is a common
occurrence, take 30 drops of gentian tincture in a glass of
water before meals to stimulate the digestive process.
To relieve discomfort, drink one cup of chamomile or
meadowsweet tea three times a day. Drink peppermint
tea if stomach ache is accompanied by flatulence.
A teaspoonful of slippery elm powder in a glass of water
is also helpful.

Thrush

Apply marigold ointment around the vagina to ease
discomfort. Wild yam, echinacea, golden seal, St John's
Wort, marigold, and buchu are often used to boost the
immune system and to assist the digestion so that thrush is
less likely to occur.

Tonsillitis

A tea of marigold, echinacea, or golden seal will help to
reduce the symptoms of tonsillitis as will a combination of
24 drops echinacea and 6 drops poke root tinctures in a
glass of water three times daily.

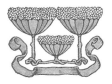

Giving up tobacco

Mix together 40 per cent tabacum
6C (homoeopathic), 10 per cent rock
rose, 30 per cent nux vom 6C
(homoeopathic), 10 per cent walnut
(Bach flower remedy), and 10 per cent
crab apple (Bach flower remedy).
Take 4 to 6 drops of this mixture under
your tongue as often as required.

Ulcers

To reduce the occurrence of mouth ulcers, take 10 to 15
drops of gentian tincture in a glass of water twice daily.
To reduce soreness and pain, gargle before meals with
equal parts of thyme, sage, and myrrh tinctures with one
teaspoon of glycerine to coat the mouth's surface. To calm
stomach ulcers, juice about one-sixth of a cabbage and
drink daily for three weeks.

Varicose veins

To improve poor circulation contributing to varicose veins,
drink a cup of ginger tea three times daily. Chili and ginger
should be added to the diet and marigold ointment
massaged into the affected area relieves itchiness and pain.
Massage strokes should be one-way strokes: upwards,
towards the heart. Never massage any veins with dark
blue lumps.

Warts

Put a dollop of comfrey or thuja ointment on the wart and
cover securely before going to bed each night until the wart
disappears.

Worms

Garlic, onions, pomegranate seeds, quassia, and wormwood
share anti-parasitic qualities, and senna, marigold, and
liquorice are excellent cleansers as are pumpkin seeds.

Herbs for Beauty

Herbal teas and lotions are a natural and economical way to pamper any body. Herbs are a natural complement to the healthy beauty basics: a well-balanced and nutritious diet, regular aerobic and non-aerobic exercise, sufficient sleep, and relaxation.

Facial steam treatment

This process induces perspiration which carries away impurities clogging the skin's pores. Herbal leaves or flowers are simmered in water to release their volatile essences and medicating, cleansing properties. Once weekly steaming is beneficial; more frequent steaming could disturb the skin's natural oil and moisture balance.

You will need:

2 tablespoons of fresh herbal leaves or flowers (or 1 tablespoon dried)

5 cups (40 fl oz/1.25 litres) water

A non-aluminum saucepan

A heat-proof mat

A standard bathtowel

Hair secured to free a thoroughly cleaned face and neck.

Slowly bring the herbs and water to the boil and simmer covered for about 3 minutes. Then move the saucepan to the heat-proof mat or pour the contents into a bowl. Hold your face about 8 inches (20 cm) from the water, enveloping your head and the saucepan with the towel. Close your eyes, turning your head slowly from side to side to allow even penetration by the herbal steam.

For fine skin or skin with visible surface veins, a 5 minute treatment is sufficient. For normal to oily skin, allow 10 minutes.

After steaming, rinse the face with warm water, pat gently with soft cotton soaked in a cold herb tea, and finally pat dry. Allow the skin to settle for one hour before going outdoors or applying cosmetics.

Suggestions for facial steams

Normal to dry skin
Chopped comfrey leaves, chopped comfrey root, and whole chamomile flowers mixed in equal quantities.

Dry, sensitive skin
Borage leaves and flowers, sorrel.

Normal to oily skins
Chopped comfrey leaves and comfrey root, chopped lemongrass, crushed fennel seeds, and crumbled lavender flowers mixed in equal quantities.

Problem skins
Chopped comfrey root, crumbled lavender flowers, and chopped lemongrass mixed in equal quantities.

For acne
Juniper or antiseptic and healing hyssop leaves or a few drops of their essential oils are recommended.

To tighten and stimulate the skin
Chopped peppermint leaves, chopped comfrey leaves, crushed aniseed, and rosemary leaves mixed in equal quantities. Also crushed bay leaves, chamomile flowers, rosemary leaves, and rose petals.

To add moisture and soothe the skin
Chopped orange peel, whole orange blossoms, chopped comfrey root, and crushed fennel seeds mixed in equal quantities.

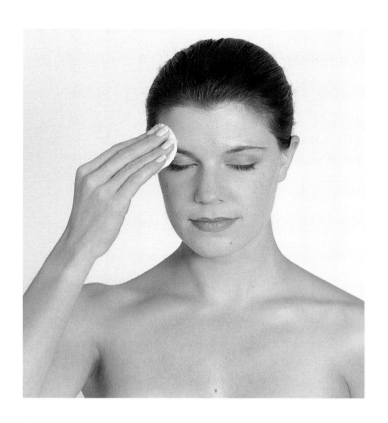

If you have broken or visible capilliaries, do not attempt a facial steam or a face pack, or subject your skin to extremes of heat and cold. Instead, try cooled, soothing herb teas made from comfrey leaves, comfrey root, chamomile flowers, or elderflowers applied to the face with absorbent cotton pads.

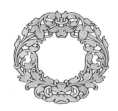

Herbal cosmetics

A herbal face mask

Fennel seed is said to smooth out lines; chamomile is astringent and anti-inflammatory; sage is cooling and astringent; elderflowers lighten and soothe the skin and are especially good for helping to fade freckles. Yogurt and honey clear and soften the skin. Fuller's earth, an absorbent clay powder, stimulates facial circulation, drawing impurities to the surface.

2 teaspoons of any of the following herbs:

fennel seeds

chamomile flowers

sage leaves

elderflowers

1 cup water

6 tablespoons plain yogurt

1 tablespoon honey

1 tablespoon Fuller's earth, available commercially

Simmer herbs in water for 15 minutes, reducing liquid to a decoction of about 1 tablespoon when strained into a clean bowl. Add yogurt, honey, and Fuller's earth. Mix well and refrigerate until cool. Cleanse face thoroughly before applying mixture lightly to face and neck with absorbent cotton pads. Rest for 15 minutes before removing mixture with cotton pads dipped in warm water or strained herbal tea of your choice and gently patting dry.

Fresh strawberry vitalizer

After cleansing the skin or after a facial steam, pulp enough strawberries to spread over face and neck, leaving the eye area clear. Rest for 20 minutes — with cotton wool pads soaked in cold, crushed fennel seed tea on your closed eyelids. Use warm water to rinse off the mask before splashing with cold water.

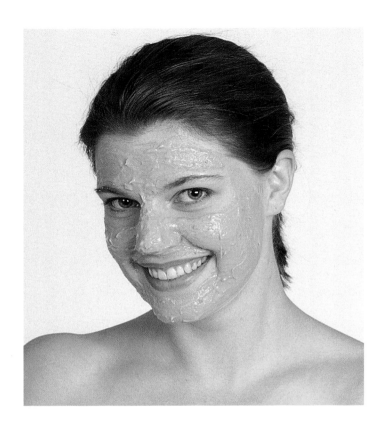

*Natural face masks
and lotions promote a dewy glow
and soft texture.*

Elderflower soother

Use this lotion to soothe and remove the redness of sunburn. Used regularly, it may help to fade freckles and give the complexion a fine-textured, soft finish. The quantity produced by the following recipe is sufficient for one week's treatment.

Pour 2 cups boiling water onto

2 tablespoons of crumbled fresh elderflowers or

1 tablespoon of fragmented dried elderflowers.

Cover and leave for at least 15 minutes before straining into a sterile container and storing in the refrigerator.

Instead of washing your face in the morning, pour some elderflower lotion into a small bowl, saturate absorbent cotton pads and apply to face and neck, allowing the lotion to dry on the skin.

Herbal aftershave

1 tablespoon chopped sage leaves

1 tablespoon chopped comfrey leaves

1 tablespoon rosemary leaves

1¹/2 cups apple cider vinegar

1¹/2 cups witchhazel

Put the herbs and vinegar into a sterile, stoppered glass jar and stand it on a sunny windowsill to infuse for 1 week. Strain, then stir in the witchhazel. Refrigerate in a sterile, airtight container.

Avocado freshener

Scoop the flesh from half an avocado and mash. Spread the pulp on the face and neck and rest for 20 minutes. Remove the moisturizing avocado with tissues, splash gently with lukewarm water and pat dry.

Avocado oil makes an excellent, everyday moisturizer for face, neck, legs and arms.

Honey and milk rejuvenator

1 cup clear honey

¹/2 cup milk

2 teaspoons rosewater

Non-aluminum saucepan

Gently warm the honey in the saucepan. Remove from heat and add milk and rosewater, stirring to combine all ingredients. Allow to cool, transfer to sterilized container and refrigerate. Before use, stir if necessary to recombine the ingredients. Pour a little lotion into a saucer. Soak absorbent cotton pads in the lotion and pat onto the face and neck. For best results, use this lotion every night and do not rinse it off until the next morning.

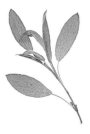

Skin washes

Soak absorbent cotton pads in cooled herbal infusions and gently pat onto the skin. For sensitive or tender skin, use a spray to administer the cooled infusion.

Comfrey leaf tea is an excellent tonic for the complexion.

Sage tea will help to close enlarged pores.

Weak horehound tea is used to treat minor skin problems.

An infusion of salad burnet, cooled and applied to the face regularly, will also help clear the skin.

Aniseed tea is said to lighten the skin.

For an effective skin-refresher and to help fade freckles, infuse some sliced horseradish root in milk or yogurt and pat onto the skin.

Greasy skin responds well to the inclusion of two cups of weak yarrow tea in the daily diet for a few weeks. Beyond that time, yarrow tea may make skin sensitive to light, so cautious use is advisable. Cooled, leftover tea can be used as a facial rinse and also helps to heal chapped hands.

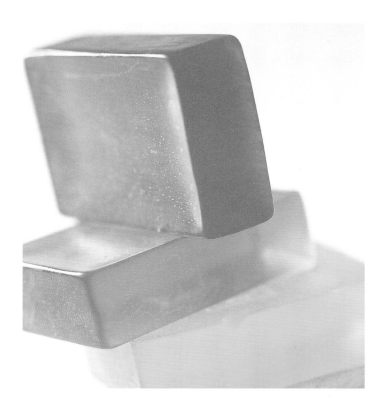

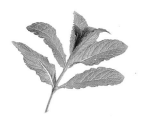

Hair treatments

Infuse rosemary, sage, and southernwood in vinegar in a stoppered bottle kept at a sunny window for one week before straining. Massage into hair and scalp before shampooing.

Infuse sage, thyme, marjoram, and balm steeped in olive oil in a stoppered bottle stored at a sunny window for one week before straining. Massage into hair and scalp before shampooing.

Shampoos and hair lotions containing pure extract of rosemary revitalize the scalp and hair and help prevent dandruff. Simmer 4 to 6 leafy rosemary stalks in a covered saucepan with 5 cups (40 fl oz/1.25 L) of water for 30 minutes. Strain and cool. Use as a final rinse after washing your hair, massaging the lotion well into the scalp.

Marjoram and sage treatments will darken brunette hair and cover grey hair

Scented baths

Gather fresh or dried herbs into a muslin or cheesecloth bag and hold under hot running water or float the sealed bag in the bath. Alternatively, make a double-strength infusion of herbal tea and add this to the bath.

Large herbal leaves, first "bruised" by rubbing with the hands to release their active essences, may be floated directly in the bath water.

Fresh or dried lavender flowers or leaves or a few drops of lavender oil infused in hot bathwater create an antiseptic bath that is especially healing to troubled skin while it soothes and refreshes the spirit.

Angelica offers fragrant relaxation.

Lemon balm cleanses and perfumes the skin and is often used in conjunction with other herbs in the bathwater.

Lovage, a deodorizing herb, may be considered as an all-over body freshening bath.

A few sprays of rosemary or drops of rosemary oil in the morning bath give an invigorating start to the day. At dusk, a rosemary bath will help revive mind and body to make the most of the evening.

Marjoram and lemon verbena are refreshing after physical exertion. Salad burnet's fresh cucumber fragrance and summer or winter savory also make stimulating baths.

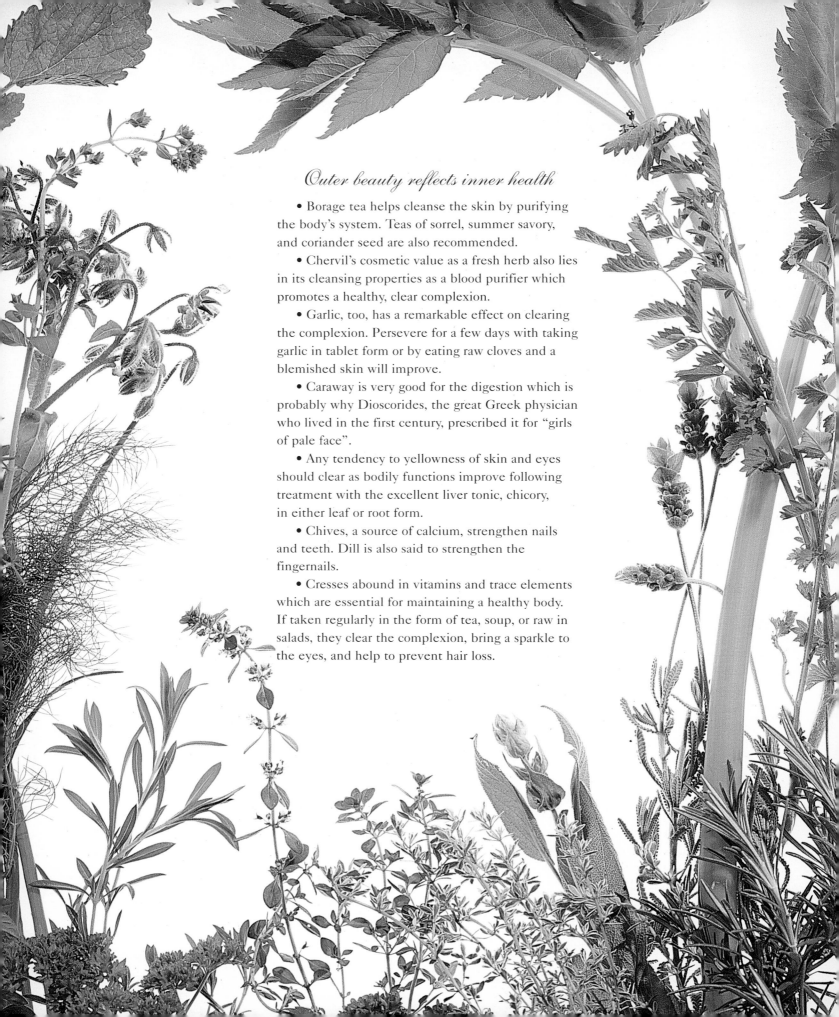

Outer beauty reflects inner health

• Borage tea helps cleanse the skin by purifying the body's system. Teas of sorrel, summer savory, and coriander seed are also recommended.

• Chervil's cosmetic value as a fresh herb also lies in its cleansing properties as a blood purifier which promotes a healthy, clear complexion.

• Garlic, too, has a remarkable effect on clearing the complexion. Persevere for a few days with taking garlic in tablet form or by eating raw cloves and a blemished skin will improve.

• Caraway is very good for the digestion which is probably why Dioscorides, the great Greek physician who lived in the first century, prescribed it for "girls of pale face".

• Any tendency to yellowness of skin and eyes should clear as bodily functions improve following treatment with the excellent liver tonic, chicory, in either leaf or root form.

• Chives, a source of calcium, strengthen nails and teeth. Dill is also said to strengthen the fingernails.

• Cresses abound in vitamins and trace elements which are essential for maintaining a healthy body. If taken regularly in the form of tea, soup, or raw in salads, they clear the complexion, bring a sparkle to the eyes, and help to prevent hair loss.

Breath-fresheners and teeth-brighteners

Infusions of lemon balm, aniseed, summer or winter savory freshen the mouth and sweeten the breath.

Spearmint, incorporated into a number of herbal toothpastes to whiten teeth and condition the gums, will also help to prevent bad breath when used to make an effective digestive tea.

To whiten the teeth, simply rub with sage leaves. To prevent the formation of dental tartar, chew strawberries.

Cooled thyme tea is an effective mouthwash and thyme is frequently an ingredient in herbal toothpastes.

Herbal beauty tips

Aloe vera
Aloe vera gel straight from the plant has a healing, smoothing, anti-wrinkling effect on the skin. It is also beneficial when rubbed into the hair and scalp.

Basil
Fresh basil leaves contribute their unique fragrance to an aromatic, body-toning massage oil when alternated with layers of coarse, fresh sea salt and cold-pressed, fine vegetable oil. This delightful concoction should be sealed in a sterile jar and stored in a cool, dark place for a few weeks before careful straining prior to use.

Chamomile
An infusion of chamomile flowers, strained, cooled and used as a hair rinse has been used for centuries to lighten the hair. Chamomile facial steams soothe and strengthen the skin. The herb is also used in facial masks, moisturizers, soaps, sunburn lotions, eye drops and footbaths.

Comfrey
Comfrey cream or ointment soothes and heals the skin. It is especially beneficial when applied overnight to the very soft tissue under the eyes. Comfrey leaves in a facial steam help tired and ageing skins. Comfrey tea helps cleanse the bloodstream and clear the complexion.

Fennel seed
A traditional ingredient of homemade herbal beauty preparations, fennel seed is said to smooth facial lines away. A strong infusion of the seed is blended with honey and buttermilk to create an excellent skin cleanser. A mild infusion of fennel seed makes an excellent skin freshener. Absorbent cotton pads saturated in the same infusion

refreshes tired eyes when rested on the closed eyelids for about 5 minutes.

Lemongrass
Lemongrass contains vitamin A and when used externally, improves the skin. When taken internally as a tea, or in tablet form, it helps to clear the complexion, giving it a fine texture and luminous glow. People with skin problems will benefit from a course of lemongrass tablets, or by drinking the tea. An extra bonus is bright, clear eyes.

Mint
Both spearmint and peppermint can be made into double-strength teas, cooled, and then used as a final rinse for conditioning oily hair. Spearmint has also been used for helping heal chapped hands. Add a few drops of essential oil of any mint or a few sprigs of fresh mint to hot bathwater for a stimulating, refreshing physical indulgence.

Parsley
Cooled parsley tea rubbed into the scalp and hair before shampooing adds shine to dark hair. The cooled tea may also be patted onto the skin as both a toner and a freshener.

Thyme
The herb is used in natural deodorants, soaps, bath salts and facial toners. Thyme may also be used in a facial steam for normal skin.

To revitalize eye area, cover with cotton pads soaked in fennel seed or peppermint tea.

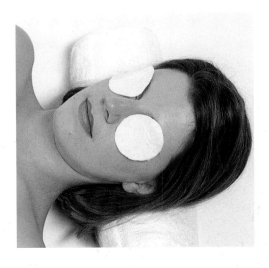

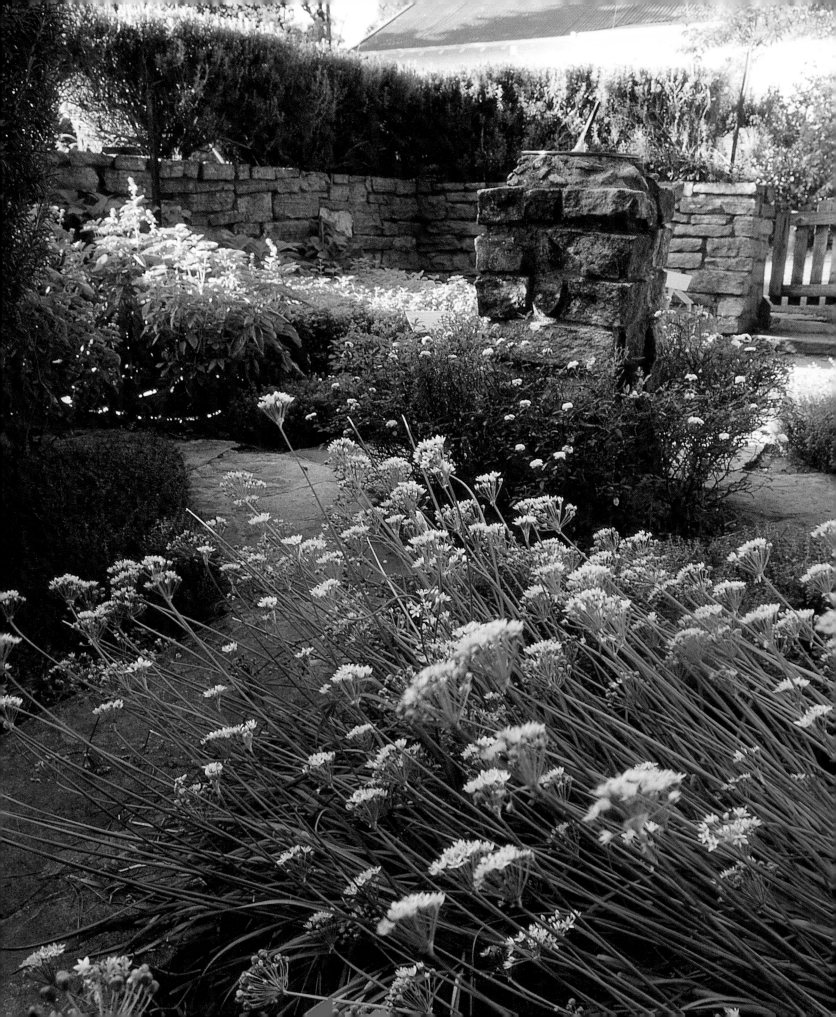

Growing Herbs

Although most herbs are available fresh-cut from stores,
and ready-made herbal products can be bought commercially,
it is handy, satisfying, and cost-effective to grow your own herbs.
A selection of culinary and healing herbs can be grown in containers,
amongst other plants in the garden, or in a special herb garden.

A simple, neat herb garden could be about 12 feet (4 metres) square, well-drained and situated in a sunny, open position. However, herbs make excellent rockery plants and also look charming when planted to form the complicated knot gardens popular in Tudor times.

Distinctive character can be bestowed on the smallest and simplest of herb gardens by the addition of a focal point such as a sundial, a statue, a pool or fountain, a birdbath or herb-seat. The latter is made of brick or stone, filled with earth, and covered with a matting scented thyme or starry-flowered lawn-chamomile.

Paths of mown grass, paving stones, pebbles, or pine bark allow easy access to herbs for harvesting or cultivating. These can be boldly incorporated in the herb garden's design by using the classic chequerboard layout, alternating pavers with herb-pockets. The beauty of this design is that it can start small but expand as desires and space permits, maintaining either the traditional square perimeter or breaking through it here and there.

Another visually delightful yet very practical and accessible herb garden design is a circular, mandala pattern, with a tendency to arrangement in fours. Buddhists regard the mandala as a symbol of the universe and use it as an aid to meditation. In the psychology of Jung, the mandala is a symbol of the wholeness of the self.

Choosing the herbs

Whatever the design, several small plants useful for edging are chives, chervil, lemon thyme, savory, bush basil, and curled parsley. Behind them, for graduated height, can be grown borage, lemon balm, sweet basil, bergamot, marjoram, French sorrel, oregano, Florentine fennel, tarragon, and dill. Some taller herbs for background planting are angelica, lovage, garlic, upright rosemary, Italian parsley, and chicory. Scented lavender or rosemary are excellent plants for surrounding a garden and may be shaped and pruned after flowering. Bay trees naturally grow to be quite large but can be kept compact with judicious pruning. Elder trees and lemon verbena trees may be placed as sheltering and protective guardians within your garden.

You might also like to select your plantings to create a theme for your herb garden. A perfumed herb garden could be grown with herbs of a variety of scent types: sweet, invigorating, or soothing. Culinary herbs might be your preference or you might choose to concentrate on those which can be used for medicinal and cosmetic purposes as well as culinary ones. Those with an interest in astrology might choose to plant some of the herbs which the ancients assigned to particular planets. Jupiter's herbs include agrimony, balm, borage, hyssop, and sage. Under Mars are basil, chives, tarragon and wormwood. For Mercury, plant caraway, dill, fennel, lavender, savory, marjoram, oregano, and parsley. The Sun signs could grow a small bay tree, salad burnet, chamomile, marigold, rosemary, or rue. Venus indicates catnip, the mints, mugwort, tansy, violet, and yarrow.

Because of the part herbs play in Mediterranean mythology, the horticultural myth has arisen that they prefer harsh conditions. This is no more true of herbs than it is for most plants. Herb gardeners, too, need to provide the majority of their plants with access to sunlight, good shelter, and healthy, well-drained soil. The ideal soil is crumbly and slightly grainy. It won't compact into a hard mass like clay, nor run through your fingers like sand. However, herbs generally do not like soil enriched with fertilizers and manures although garden compost is always helpful and before planting, herb beds should be prepared by digging in plenty of leaf mould and mushroom or household compost. While extra compost will counter a too sandy or light soil, a small amount of coarse river sand will lighten heavy soil.

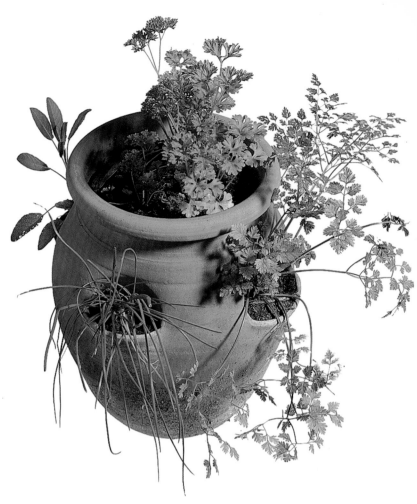

Herbs in containers

If treated as indoor plants, herbs will become leggy and yellow, then die. But they are easily grown in containers placed on a balcony, window ledge, or anywhere they have access to plenty of sun and air.

Good drainage, too, is essential to most herbs, so when selecting a pot, make sure that it has holes in the base to allow excess water to escape. Covering the drainage holes with a base layer of uneven pebbles will retain soil but allow water through.

Terracotta containers dry out quickly on dry days unless equipped with saucers filled with water which the porous pot will absorb to keep itself and its plant cool and moist.

Trough-shaped pots in various materials and sizes often fit snugly on a window ledge and many container gardeners choose a strawberry pot or jar with five or six lipped holes in the sides, each planted with herbs.

To plant a strawberry pot with herbs, place one large or several smaller, uneven stones above the drainage hole in the base. Then fill the jar with potting mixture to the level of the lowest lipped holes. Plant a herb seedling down through the pot's main open diameter, gently manipulating the foliage through one of the side holes with the roots

within. Fill the pot with soil level to the next aperture and repeat the process as before. When the top has been reached, plant with one last herb, leaving about 1 inch (2 cm) between the last layer of soil and the rim of the pot to allow for watering. To water a strawberry or herb jar, fill the pot with water to the very top and let it soak through. Repeat about three times to ensure that the lowest layer of plants receive sufficient moisture. Never fill a strawberry jar with soil and sow seeds in the lipped holes because they will wash out when watering.

Hanging baskets can be ideal for herbs which will thrive suspended from a beam or window architrave in the right spot. Consider a terracotta one, with or without strawberry slots, or a wire frame lined with bark or other fibrous material. Wicker lobster pots, woven in varying shapes and sizes and equipped with chains for hanging them, are highly prized as attractive and practical herb planters when lined with damp newspaper or some other organic material to allow the potting soil to drain but not to spill through the basket weave.

For larger spaces, large tubs, perhaps wooden wine barrels cut in half, will allow you to enjoy the exuberant growth habit of many herbs.

Small-growing culinary herbs with compact root systems, such as thyme, chives, marjoram, sage, oregano, parsley, and chervil, can be planted fairly close together and still flourish. A trough approximately 2 feet (60 cm) long and 8 inches (20 cm) wide will comfortably hold five herbs, especially if they are staggered. A shallow pot of 16 inches (40 cm) diameter holds up to seven plants.

Tips for cultivating herbs

• Regularly remove old growth and dead wood to promote new growth and keep your herbs looking attractively vigorous.

• When planting out potted herbs, first moisten the soil so that it will cling to the roots and then tap out gently.

• With the exception of parsley and chives, herbs develop a stronger flavor in relatively infertile soils, so don't be tempted to lavish them with masses of compost. Similarly, they generally prefer dry feet, so don't overwater or plant in poorly-drained soils. The exception is watercress which, as its name suggests, thrives in waterlogged positions.

• Mint, with its invasive root system, is better grown in its own pot, otherwise it will take over the whole container, outgrowing and limiting any companion herbs.

Seeds

• Pots or tubs should be filled to about 1/2 inch (1 cm) from the top to allow for easy watering.

• Seed boxes should be placed on a level surface and the seeds sown along furrows.

• When covering seed in a box, the soil should be rubbed through the hands and any hard lumps discarded before the fine, powdery seed-raising mixture is firmly and evenly pressed level.

• Keep the seedbed moist at all times. If soil is dry for just a short time, germination may cease.

Herbs from cuttings

• Use a sharp knife, scissors, or garden sheers to take cuttings from parent plants just below a leaf node.

• About one third of the foliage should be left at the top, cut leaves off or pull them in upwards to avoid stem damage.

• To prevent cuttings from wilting, keep them in water, or wrapped in a damp cloth until ready to plant.

• Use a knitting needle or a skewer to make a hole to receive a cutting. Never just push a trimmed stem into its potting medium.

• Dip the moist, lower 1/2 inch (1 cm) of each cutting into a suitable cutting powder, shake off excess, and insert one-third of the stem into the potting mix, covering at least two leaf nodes if possible.

• If using sand as a potting medium to strike cuttings, use coarse river sand. Beach sand is too fine and salty.

• When cuttings are first put in sand, flood with water so the sand will pack tightly around the cuttings and water daily to keep sand moist at all times.

• To help cuttings make roots in cool climates, place them in a glasshouse, or if this is not possible, lay a sheet of glass over a box, making sure the glass is painted with whitewash to prevent the plants being scorched by the sun's rays.

• Rooted cuttings can be transplanted from sand directly into soil, but it is best to first transplant them to small separate pots in semi-shade for several weeks.

Herbal insect repellents

A strong wormwood tea, cooled, and poured on the tracks of slugs and snails in spring and autumn is an effective natural deterrent.

This garlic garden spray is another organic repellent for aphids, snails, cabbage moth, caterpillars and mosquitoes, especially effective when used every 2 weeks.

You'll need these ingredients:

3 big cloves unpeeled garlic

6 tablespoons medicinal paraffin oil

1 tablespoon grated oil-based soap

2 cups (16 fl oz/500ml) hot water

To make the spray, roughly chop garlic, blend it with paraffin oil, and leave the pulp in a covered bowl for 48 hours. Dissolve grated soap in hot water and add it to the garlic and oil pulp. When cool, strain the mixture into screw-top jars and store in refrigerator. Use 2 tablespoons of this solution in 8 cups (64 fl oz/2 litres) of water.

Drying Herbs

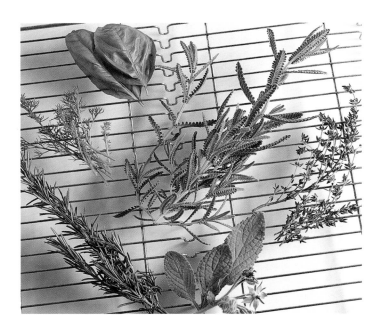

For efficient, natural drying, branchlets of herbs can be laid on airy, mesh trays in a warm, dry atmosphere out of direct sunlight and where air circulates freely. Spreading herbs on clean newspaper and leaving in a dry but shady area is also an excellent method. If the leaves are the type to retain moisture, prevent mold or mildew from forming by placing them so that they do not touch each other.

Never dry foliage in the sun because it will destroy the natural, concentrated essences. However, if herb flowerheads such as fennel and dill are to be dried for seed, a final sun-drying is excellent. Drying in a microwave oven can be successful and a warm (not hot) conventional oven is acceptable, but leafy stalks should be watched for signs of sticking, shrivelling, or burning and constantly turned.

Drying times are variable, depending on temperature, humidity, and the season. However, a dependable sign of thorough dryness is brittleness.

Drying herbs in a microwave oven

Microwave drying is a very efficient and quick method of dehydrating freshly picked herbs. Place them on absorbent paper to absorb excess moisture and microwave them for 30 seconds. Continue in 30 second intervals until the first sign of crispness is evident. Then reduce microwaving to 15 second intervals. Most herbs seem to dry in about 3 to 4 minutes, although chervil takes as little as 1 minute to dry, and chives a little more than 4 minutes. Because herbs do vary in drying time, even 15 seconds could be crucial.

Storing

When foliage and flowers are brittle, strip remaining foliage by hand. Store the dried foliage in clean, dry, preferably dark glass containers, labelled and dated. Clear glass containers should be stored away from light, not on a bright kitchen bench or window ledge.

Washed sprays of fresh herbs, as well as chopped fresh herbs, can be wrapped in foil or plastic and stored in the refrigerator for a week. They may also be frozen for up to three weeks — wash, chop finely, and freeze in ice cube trays with a little water. When needed, defrost the frozen herbs, or use them without thawing.

If you are drying herbs for their aromatic foliage, a general rule is to gather them on a dry day, as early as possible in the morning once any dew has evaporated, and before the heat of the sun extracts most of the active oils in the foliage. Drying concentrates these essential oils.

Unless herbs have been sprayed with insecticide, don't wash the plants. This way you'll retain all the natural essences clinging to the surface of their foliage and avoid triggering the growth of mildew.

Drying herbs

The simplest way to dry herbs is to bundle them together neatly in bunches, tie with string, and hang them upside down in an airy but dark and dust-free place. Steamy rooms such as kitchens do not make good herbal drying rooms. To protect against dust and insects, provide protective darkness yet still allow airflow, punch holes in a paper bag, place it over the foliage and tie around the stalks before hanging. This way, too, as the foliage dries and falls, it is collected in the bottom of the bag.

Herbs and Their Botanical Names

Agrimony *Agrimonia eupatoria*
Aloe *Aloe vera*
Angelica *Angelica archangelica*
Aniseed *Pimpinella anisum*
Balm *Melissa officinalis*
Basil, Sweet *Ocimum basilicum*
Bay leaf *Laurus nobilis*
Bearberry (also uva ursi)
    Arctostaphylos uva ursi
Bergamot *Monarda didyma*
Bittersweet *Solanum dulcamara*
Black cohosh *Cimicifuga racemosa*
Boneset *Eupatorium perfoliatum*
Borage *Borago officinalis*
Buchu *Agathosma betulina*
Burdock *Arctium lappa*
Caraway *Carum carvi*
Cascara sagrada *Rhamnus purshiana*
Catnip *Nepeta cataria*
Cayenne *Capsicum frutescens minimum*
Celandine *Chelidonium maju*s
Celery *Apium graveolens*
Chamomile *Matricaria chamomilla* or *recutita*
    (German); *Anthemis nobilis* (Roman)
Chaste tree *Vitex agnus-castus*
Chervil *Anthriscus cerefolium*
Chickweed *Stellaria media*
Chicory root *Chicorum intybus*
Chili *Capsicum frutescens annuum*
Chive *Allium schoenoprasum*
Cinnamon *Cinnamomum zeylanicum*
Clivers (also cleavers) *Galium aparine*
Coltsfoot *Tussilago farfara*
Comfrey *Symphytum officinale*
Coriander seed *Coriandrum sativum*
Corn silk *Zea mays*
Cramp bark *Viburnum opulus*
Cranesbill *Geranium maculatum*
Cress *Nastertium officinale*
Damiana *Turnera aphrodisiaca*
Dandelion *Taraxacum officinale*
Dill *Anethum graveolens*
Echinacea *Echinacea angustifolia*
Elder *Sambucus nigra*

Elecampane *Inula helenium*
Evening primrose oil *Oenothera biennis*
Eyebright *Euphrasia officinalis*
False unicorn root *Chamaelirium luteum*
Fennel, florentine *Foeniculum vulgare dulce*
Feverfew *Chrysanthemum parthenium*
Fringetree *Chionanthus virginicus*
Garlic *Allium sativum*
Gentian *Gentiana lutea*
Ginger *Zingiber officinale*
Ginseng *Panax ginseng*
Golden rod *Solidago virgauria*
Golden seal *Hydrastis canadensis*
Grindelia *Grindelia camporum*
Guaiacum *Guaiacum officinale*
Hawthorn berries *Crataegus oxyacanthoides*
Hops *Humulus lupulus*
Horehound *Murrubium vulgare*
Horse-chestnut *Aesculus hippocastanum*
Horseradish *Cochlearis armoracia*
Hyssop *Hyssopus officinalis*
Jamaican dogwood *Piscidia erythrina*
Juniper *Juniperus communus*
Lavender *Lavandula augustifolia*;
    Lavandula spica;Lavandula officinalis
Lemon balm *Melissa officinalis*
Lemon verbeena *Aloysia triphylla*
Lemongrass *Cymbopogon citratus*
Lime flower (also linden blossom)
    Tilia europea
Linden (also lime flower) *Tilia europea*
Liquorice *Glycyrrhiza glabra*
Lobelia *Lobelia inflata*
Lovage *Levisticum officinale*
Marigold *Calendula officinalis*
Marjoram *Origanum majorana*
Marshmallow *Althaea officinalis*
Meadowsweet *Filipendula ulmaria*
Mint *Mentha arvenis* (field mint);
    Mentha piperita (peppermint);
    Mentha spicata (spearmint);
    Mentha pulegium (pennyroyal)
Motherwort *Leonurus cardiaca*
Mugwort *Artemisia vulgaris*

Myrrh *Commiphora molmol*
Nettle *Urtica dioica*
Oak bark *Quercus robur*
Oats *Avena sativa*
Orange blossoms *Citrus reticulata*
Oregano *Origanum vulgare*
Parsley *Petroselinum crispum*
Passionflower *Passiflora incarnata*
Pelargonium gravolens *Geranium*
Plantain *Plantago major*
Poke root *Phytolacca decandra*
Prickly ash *Zanthoxylum americanum*
Quassia *Picrasma excelsa*
Rasberry leaf *Rubus idaeus*
Red clover *Trifolium pratense*
Rhubarb root *Rheum palmatum*
Rosehip *Rosa species*
Rosemary *Rosmarinus officinalis*
Rue *Ruta graveolens*
Sage *Salvia officinalis*
Salad Burnet *Sanguisorba minor*
Savory, summer *Satureia hortensis*
Savory, winter *Satureia montana*
Senna pods *Cassia senna*
Skullcap *Scutellaria laterifloia*
Slippery elm *Ulmus fulva*
Solanum oil *see Bittersweet*
Sorrel *Rumex scutatus*
Southernwood *Artemisia abrotanum*
St John's Wort *Hypericum perforatum*
Stinging Nettle *Urtica dioica*
Tansy *Tanacetum vulgare*
Tarragon *Artemisia dracunculus*
Thuja (also arbor vitae) *Thuja occidentalis*
Thyme *Thymus vulgaris*
Valerian *Valeriana officinalis*
Vervain *Verbena officinalis*
Wild cherry bark *Prunus serotina*
Wild yam *Dioscorea villosa*
Witchhazel *Hamamelis virginiana*
Wood betony *Stachys betonica*
Wormwood *Artemisia absinthium*
Yarrow *Achillea millefolium*
Yellow dock *Rumex crispus*

Acknowledgments

The publisher gratefully acknowledges the contribution to The Healing Art of Herbs
of John and Rosemary Hemphill
by allowing their many books on herbs and herbalism to be used as references for the text.
Their caring interest in the production of this title is warmly appreciated.

Sincere thanks also to Toni Eatts
for her contributions to the chapters Herbalism in History, Chinese Herbal Medicine and
Bach Flower Remedies. A special thanks to herbalist Robyn Kirby for her contribution to the chapter
Healing with Herbs and thanks also to Katie Davis for her assistance with that chapter.

Thanks to Christine Falvey for her research, writing and editing.

For photograph (page 11): Australian Picture Library/ET Archive
For photograph (page 18): AKG London/Erich Lessing
For photographs of herbs: John Hemphill
For photographs (pages 2, 14-15, 17, 21, 39-42, 45, 47-55, 62):
Photographer — André Martin, Stylist — Mary-Anne Danaher
Glass teapot supplied by Penelope Sach, Woollahra NSW Australia.
Also thanks to The Fragrant Garden, Erina NSW Australia.

Published by Lansdowne Publishing Pty Ltd
Level 5, 70 George Street, Sydney, NSW 2000, Australia
Chief Executive Publisher: Jane Curry
Publishing Manager: Deborah Nixon
Production Manager: Sally Stokes
Project Co-ordinator: Kirsten Tilgals
Project Assistant: Amalia Matheson
Designer: Michelle Wiener

First published in 1996
© Copyright: Lansdowne Publishing Pty Ltd

Set in Caslon 540 Roman on Quark Xpress
Printed in Singapore by Tien Wah Press (Pte) Ltd

National Library of Australia Cataloguing-in-Publication Data
The healing art of herbs.
ISBN 1 86302 464 6.
1. Herbs - Therapeutic use.
615.321